The One-week Baby Sleep Solution

Your 7-day plan for a
good night's sleep – for baby
and you!

Gina Ford

Vermilion
LONDON

1 3 5 7 9 10 8 6 4 2

Vermilion, an imprint of Ebury Publishing,
20 Vauxhall Bridge Road,
London SW1V 2SA

Vermilion is part of the Penguin Random House group of companies whose
addresses can be found at global.penguinrandomhouse.com

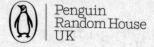

Penguin
Random House
UK

First published in the United Kingdom by Vermilion in 2018

www.penguin.co.uk

A CIP catalogue record for this book is available from the British Library

ISBN 9781785040764

Printed and bound in Great Britain by Clays Ltd, St Ives PLC

Penguin Random House is committed to a sustainable future for our
business, our readers and our planet. This book is made from Forest
Stewardship Council® certified paper.

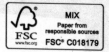

Contents

Acknowledgements

I would like a very special thank you to my editor Samantha Jackson who is the inspiration behind this book. Also to my publisher Rebecca Smart, along with editors Julia Kellaway, Louise Francis and Emma Owen and the rest of the team at Penguin Random House, who continue to give me much encouragement and support.

A very special thank you to the Contentedbaby. com team, editor Kate Brian, Sofiah Macleod, Alison Jermyn and Christel Davidson, for all their wonderful work on the website and also their constant support and encouragement with the writing of my books. Also to Rory Jenkins of Embado.com, whose technical skills have helped create an amazing website which reaches parents across five continents.

Finally, I would like to say thank you to the thousands of parents whom I have worked with through my consultancy service over the last 18 years. Your feedback of how the CLB routines have worked for you has helped me hugely with this book and your loving supportive messages mean more than you will ever know. Special love and thanks to you all and to your contented babies.

Introduction

Over the years I have worked with many thousands of parents, and have helped them find solutions to the challenges they were having with their babies and toddlers. My first book, *The Contented Little Baby Book* (published in 1999), was based on my experiences of working with over 300 babies and their families. Since then I have advised thousands more parents through my consultancy work and the Contented Baby website, www.contentedbaby.com, which I set up to help and support parents as they navigated their way through those early months. Through this direct contact I have become familiar with the most common problems new parents experience, and I know how tired and anxious mums and dads can become when their baby is not sleeping well.

Sleep is probably the most misunderstood and confusing aspect of parenthood. The misconception is that for the first few weeks all the baby will do is feed and sleep. While many do, the fact that that there are now literally hundreds of sleep consultants in the United Kingdom is proof that a great many do not. If your newborn or young baby is one of the latter – tense, fretful and difficult to settle – please take heart, as this need not be a reflection of your baby's future sleep habits.

There is much conflicting advice from childcare experts on how to tackle sleep problems. The majority of experts advise parents with very young babies who are waking up several times a night to wait until the baby is six months old before attempting to resolve the problem. My own personal view is that the longer parents put off trying to resolve excessive night-time waking, the harder it will be to solve problems further down the line.

If your baby has got into a routine of excessive night-time waking or has developed the wrong sleep associations, then the practical advice in this book will help you to instil better sleeping habits in your child. As long as you are prepared to be consistent and persistent, there are many solutions that will help you establish a good sleeping pattern for your child.

Gina

1

Understanding your Baby's Sleep

Before trying to implement the plans in this book, it is very important that you have a basic understanding of the different stages of sleep that babies go through. Filmed research shows that all babies come into a light sleep several times a night, some even waking up fully for short spells. When the wakings are not due to genuine hunger, the research shows that the babies who have learned to self-settle will get themselves back to sleep fairly quickly. Babies who have been rocked, patted or fed to get them to sleep are usually unable to settle themselves to sleep without the attentions that they associate with going to sleep.

Once the wrong sleep associations are created it can be very difficult for a baby to sleep for a longer stretch. A baby who is always rocked, fed or given a dummy to get to sleep will be much more likely to continue to wake several times a night, long after the age when he needs a milk feed to get him through the night (see box on page 7 for more on this). Because he will naturally come into a light sleep several times a night, he will more than likely need the same comfort to get him back to sleep at each cycle.

SLEEP CYCLES

Sleep is divided into rapid eye movement (REM) sleep, usually referred to as active (or light) sleep, and non-REM sleep, usually referred to as quiet (or deep) sleep. Unlike adults and older babies, who start out in non-REM sleep, a newborn baby goes straight into REM sleep when he first drifts off. During this active sleep, his breathing becomes irregular, his body may twitch or jerk, his eyelids will flicker and his eyes appear to roll. He may even smile or frown. His body uses more oxygen and energy during this cycle than during non-REM sleep. A baby who has gone full term will spend 50 per cent of his sleep cycle in REM sleep.

A premature baby will spend about 80 per cent in REM sleep. The rest of the sleep cycle is spent in non-REM sleep.

During non-REM sleep the baby's breathing will be slow and regular. There are no eye movements and only the occasional twitch or jerk of the body. This calm sleep cycle allows the baby's mind and body to recharge, enabling him to cope with his next awake period. Research shows us that this deep sleep is essential for the healthy development of a baby's mental and physical growth.

As Dr Richard Ferber, one of America's leading authorities in the field of children's sleep problems, explains in his book *Solve Your Child's Sleep Problems*, non-REM sleep is well developed at birth but has not evolved into the four distinct stages experienced by older children and adults. It is not until around the second month that a sequence of non-REM sleep stages begins to develop. By three months a baby will first enter sleep in stage one of non-REM – a drowsy sleep – then quickly pass into stage two – a light sleep – before reaching stages three and four – very deep sleep. The whole cycle lasts around 40 minutes in babies and for toddlers it is around 60 minutes.

I have observed that it is between the ages of eight and twelve weeks that many parents begin to experience problems with their baby's daytime sleep, as the different stages of non-REM sleep begin to develop. During the first few weeks, the majority of babies will tend to fall asleep easily – often in their baby seat or in their pram or buggy – and frequently sleep for several hours at a time. Unfortunately, as the baby's sleep cycle develops into more distinct stages of light and deep sleep, he will often find it more difficult to settle back to sleep after the 40–50-minute sleep cycle if he is used to sleeping in a bright and busy daytime atmosphere. As the day progresses, the baby gets more and more irritable, and by late afternoon he is often very overtired and fights sleep even more. Parents who don't realise that this fractious behaviour is caused by poor quality daytime sleep resort to feeding, rocking, patting, etc. to help their baby get back to sleep when he has come into his light sleep. What starts out as a daytime sleep problem soon also becomes a night-time problem. A baby who needs assistance to return to sleep when he comes into a light sleep during the day will more likely than not come to need the same help at night.

Because all babies will come into a light sleep several times a night once they have developed an adult sequence of sleep cycles, a problem can soon evolve. This can often mean several wakings a night for parents for many months and sometimes even years.

When will my baby be able to sleep through the night?

The age that a baby can sleep a longer spell in the night without needing a feed is very individual, but a baby who has gone full term and is gaining a good amount of weight each week can usually start to sleep for one longer spell of four or more hours in the night by the time he reaches one month. As the baby grows he should gradually, over the weeks and months, start to extend the length of time he sleeps, until he is going around ten to twelve hours at night at six months with a sleepy feed around 10/11pm in the evening or perhaps around 5/6am in the morning.

Of course there are many babies who may continue to need feeds in the night until they are a year old if all of their nutritional needs are not being met during the day. The most important thing that I stress to parents is that the aim in the early days should not be to push their baby through the night as quickly as possible without a feed, but to ensure that, as their baby grows, the daytime feeds are increased accordingly, so that the need to feed in the night decreases naturally. It is much better to feed your baby in the night for a little longer, and allow him to self-settle after a feed, than to try to skip feeds by offering a dummy or rocking and patting your baby back to sleep when he wakes in the night.

DAYTIME SLEEP

Research confirms what I have always believed: poor quality daytime sleep can affect not only the baby's mental development but also his ability to sleep well at night. Dr Marc Weissbluth, a leading researcher, paediatrician and founder of the Sleep Disorders Center, Children's Memorial Hospital, Chicago, and the Northwestern Children's Practice, says in his book *Healthy Sleep Habits, Happy Child*: 'Napping is one of the health habits that sets the stage for good overall sleep.' He explains that a nap offers a break from stimuli and allows the baby or child to recharge for further activity. Many other experts are in agreement that naps are essential to a baby's brain development and to helping establish long-term healthy sleep patterns. John Herman, PhD, infant sleep expert and Associate Professor of Psychology and Psychiatry at the University of Texas, says: 'If activities are being scheduled to the detriment of sleep, it's a mistake. Parents should remember that everything else in a baby's life should come after sleeping and eating.' Charles Schaefer, PhD, an American professor of psychology, supports this research and says: 'Naps structure the day, shape both the baby's and the mother's moods and offer the only opportunity for Mum to relax or accomplish a few tasks.' Although babies do vary in the amount of sleep they require, it is important that you have a clear understanding of how much sleep they need. The total amount of daily sleep your baby or toddler has between 7am and 7pm (depending on when you start your day) will play a big part in how well he sleeps at night. Listed below is an approximate guide to the number of hours of daytime sleep a baby needs:

Birth to four weeks	5 to 5½ hours
Four to eight weeks	4 to 4½ hours
Eight to twelve weeks	3½ hours
Three to six months	3 hours
Six to twelve months	2 to 3 hours

The timing of his naps is also important if overtiredness is to be avoided. Allowing a baby to have too much sleep later in the day is often the reason a baby does not settle well at bedtime. Research shows that the best time for the longest nap of the day is between 12 noon and 2pm, as this coincides with a baby's natural dip in alertness. A nap at this time will be deeper and more refreshing than a nap that starts later in the day. This further supports my view of the importance of daytime sleep being established at the right time.

Sleep required during the first year

Age	Daytime sleep 7am–7pm	Night-time sleep 7pm–7am	Total hours of sleep a day	Nap time
0–1			15½–16 hrs	5–5½ hrs
1–2			15 hrs	4–4½ hrs
2–3			14½ hrs	3½ hrs
3–4			14½ hrs	3 hrs
4–6			15 hrs	3 hrs
6–9			14½–15 hrs	2½–3 hrs
9–12			14–14½ hrs	2–2½ hrs

Morning nap

During the first week or two most newborns will only manage to stay awake for an hour or so at a time, and most of this time is taken up with feeding and changing. Between the second and fourth week they will usually be managing to stay awake properly for one to one and a half hours, although some very wakeful babies may manage to stay awake for up to two hours. The important thing to remember during the very early days is never to let your baby stay awake longer than two hours. If a baby stays awake longer than two hours he will often become overtired and fight sleep when you try to put him down for a nap. Overtiredness is one of the main causes of very young babies not settling well at nap times, and care should be taken that this does not happen (for more on overtiredness, see page 19).

By the time babies reach two months, providing they're sleeping well at night, it is likely that they will manage to stay awake nearer to two hours before needing their morning nap. A typical pattern may be that when they first wake in the morning, they will stay awake for a full two hours, then after the first nap of the day they may only manage to stay awake for one and a half hours. The important thing is to watch for your baby's cues as to when he is sleepy (see box below) and ensure that he is well fed and settled in his bed before he becomes overtired.

Signs your baby is ready to sleep

- He starts to yawn – not just once but two or three times
- His eyes start to open and close quite rapidly
- He pulls his head to one side as if trying to root for a feed
- His body becomes tense; some babies also arch their backs
- He starts grizzling or crying very suddenly
- Older babies may pull at their ears or start to suck their fingers

By the time they reach six-seven months, the majority of babies can stay awake for between two and two and a half hours, provided they're sleeping well in the night. If you are starting your day at 7am, your baby should be woken from his morning nap no later than 10am if you want him to sleep for a longer time at midday, even if this means he has a slightly shorter morning nap.

Between nine and twelve months most babies will cut right back on their morning nap, cutting it out altogether somewhere between 12 and 15 months. In my previous books I have said that the morning nap is usually dropped between 12 and 18 months, but over the last ten years I have noticed a huge link between the morning nap and early-morning waking and night-waking problems with toddlers. The link being that nearly all who slept well during the first year but then went on to experience sleeping problems were still having a morning nap. I now recommend that parents should gradually push the morning nap to later and reduce it somewhere between nine and twelve months, therefore preparing to drop it somewhere between 12 and 15 months. (See the box opposite for a detailed plan on how to eliminate the morning nap.)

Eliminating the morning nap

If your baby is over nine months and showing signs of waking earlier, not being ready for his morning nap, or reducing his lunchtime nap (all signs that a change in sleeping needs is imminent), I would suggest the following tips to help him gradually drop his morning nap altogether:

- Gradually push the morning nap on from 9.30am so that your baby is going down nearer to 9.45–10am. Once he is happily going through to this time, gradually reduce the length of the nap to 15 minutes. You can then push the lunchtime nap on to nearer 12.45pm and allow a nap of no more than two hours.
- If your baby is showing signs of not being ready to sleep at 9.45–10am, do not be tempted to drop the morning nap as doing it too early means that his lunchtime nap could come too soon, resulting in him going to bed in the evening either over-tired or early.

- Keep pushing your baby's morning nap on until he manages to get close to 11am, then allow a nap of five to ten minutes. Once he is managing to get through to 12.45–1pm for his lunchtime nap with only this short nap, you should be able to cut it out altogether and get him through to around 12.15–12.30pm for his nap, which would then be increased to two hours.

- If you find that your baby is becoming too tired to eat a proper lunch, you can always bring his lunch forward slightly for a short period until his body clock adjusts to the new nap times. I usually find that once they have had lunch they perk up enough to get through to 12.15–12.30pm.

Lunchtime/middle-of-the-day nap

A baby under one month is usually ready for this nap one to one and a half hours after the time he wakes from his morning nap, but by the time he reaches two to three months he can usually make it to two hours. Ideally, this should be the longest nap of the day, as research shows that a nap between 12 noon and 2pm coincides with the baby's natural dip in alertness.

Depending on how well the baby has slept at his morning nap, this nap usually lasts between two and two and a half hours, gradually reducing to around two hours by the time the baby is six months old. At around one year this longer nap may be cut back to one and a half hours if the baby is still having a full 45-minute nap in the morning, although it may lengthen again to two hours if the morning nap is cut right back or dropped altogether. At one year the length of the lunchtime nap is determined by how well the baby is sleeping at night. Some babies who are sleeping twelve hours at night will continue to need two hours' sleep at lunchtime, while others, if they are waking earlier in the morning, will need to have their lunchtime nap cut back.

The majority of babies will continue to need a nap in the middle of the day until they are at least two years of age, with the length of the nap again depending on how well they're sleeping at night. Babies who are starting to wake earlier in the morning or are starting to wake in the middle of the night may need to have their lunchtime nap cut down or cut out altogether. This can happen anywhere between 18 months and 3 years of age, depending on the child's individual needs.

Late afternoon nap

If a baby sleeps well at the two earlier naps of the day, this should be the shortest of the three naps. By the time they reach 12 weeks, the majority of babies who have slept well at lunchtime will only need a very short nap of 10–20 minutes in order to revive them enough for the bath and bedtime routine. This nap is usually dropped somewhere between three and four months of age, provided they're sleeping well at their lunchtime nap. If a baby is having less than two hours at lunchtime, he may continue to need 10–15 minutes in the late afternoon until nearer nine months of age.

Overtiredness

How long a baby can stay awake depends on the age of the baby and varies from baby to baby, but if a young baby is kept awake too long, he will become overtired. Once this happens the build-up of the stress hormones cortisol and adrenaline take over the body. This prevents him from drifting off to sleep naturally and leaves him in a stressed state of neither being able to stay awake happily or settle to sleep happily. It can often take several hours before the baby will eventually fall asleep, exhausted. With very young babies, by the time they do eventually fall asleep, they will often wake up again after a very short time because their next feed is due, and because they are so overtired it can often take a further couple of hours before the baby settles back to sleep again. Within a very short period of time a pattern of difficulty in settling to sleep and staying asleep for any length of time has emerged.

Trying to break a pattern of overtiredness is not easy once it has become established. If you feel your baby is showing signs of overtiredness, or if overtiredness has already set in, the following guidelines should help you break the vicious cycle:

- Wake your baby up at the same time every morning and start to wind him down earlier than his nap time so that he does not become overtired.
- Watch for signs that he is getting tired, and ensure that you start the wind-down time for his nap well in advance so you do not miss his cues.
- Keep things calm and build in plenty of wind-down time before naps and bedtime. Do not overstimulate your baby with lots of talking or cot mobiles and toys at bedtime. Also watch how long you keep him in his bath; with babies under six months, ten minutes is normally more than enough if you do not want to miss the window of opportunity for settling him to sleep.

- Your baby should be settled in his bed when he is sleepy but still awake. Although all babies are different, the chart on page 11 will give you an idea of approximate times and lengths of naps at the different ages during the first year.

- The times and length of naps are very important. If you allow your baby to have too much sleep in the morning, it could reduce the length of his afternoon naps, resulting often in two short naps, which then results in him becoming overtired at bedtime.

- Once your baby is over six months and sleeping in his own room, make sure that lights are kept dim and that blackout blinds are used during the day and in the evenings during the light nights, as darkness sends a signal to the baby's brain that it is time for sleep.

For more on overtiredness, see page 42 for babies from birth to six months and page 63 for babies from six to twelve months.

ESTABLISHING A BEDTIME ROUTINE

The majority of experts agree that a good bedtime routine is important for young babies and children. However, there is much disagreement over the age at which parents should start a bedtime routine and what it should consist of. Somewhere between the ages of six and twelve weeks seems to be the time most experts think you can start to establish regular times for a bath, feed and then settling the baby in his bed.

My own view is that the sooner a bedtime routine is established, the less likely the parents are to encounter problems trying to settle their baby. When I worked as a maternity nurse I established a routine in the very early days, usually around the fifth day, when the mother's milk had come in. I believe that this is one of the reasons I rarely had to deal with a crying baby in the evening. Of course there are times in the early days when a young baby will not immediately fall asleep, but if you are consistent in how you try to settle him, a pattern should very quickly emerge where he settles quickly and easily between 6.30 and 7pm. This will have a knock-on effect on what happens later and in the middle of the night. A baby who feeds and settles well in the early evening and sleeps until his next feed is due is much more likely to feed well at the last feed of the night, which should come at around 10 or 11pm. This is particularly true of breast-fed babies, as the time the baby sleeps in the evening allows the mother to have a meal and a good rest, which will help ensure that she has time to produce enough milk for a good feed last thing at night. A young baby who has a good last feed is much more likely only to wake up once in the night and then settle quickly, because again the mother will have had sufficient rest to produce enough milk for a full feed.

Regardless of whether he is bottle- or breast-fed, if a baby gets into the habit of catnapping in the early evening, he will more than likely get into the habit of feeding little and often. When the parents attempt to offer him a late feed before they go to bed, it is very unlikely that he will take a full feed, particularly if he has fed within the last couple of hours. If he doesn't feed well at the late feed, or refuses it altogether, he can end up waking up a further one or two times after midnight with a genuine need to feed. This then has a negative knock-on effect on daytime feeds. A pattern of excessive night-time feeding is very quickly established, and for a breast-feeding mother this can have dire consequences as tiredness sets in and the milk supply is greatly reduced.

If you wish to avoid a pattern of unsettled evenings and excessive waking in the middle of the night, I would strongly advise that you establish a bedtime routine as soon as possible. The following chapter deals in detail with unsettled evenings and offers several simple solutions to help your baby to settle well.

2

Unsettled Evenings

Regardless of whether you are parents of a very young baby or one several months old, if bedtimes have become a battle, please be reassured that by following the simple advice outlined in this chapter, you will be able to resolve this problem very quickly and, most importantly, without lots of tears.

BIRTH TO SIX MONTHS

I have listed below the main reasons why young babies do not settle in the evening. It may be that only one or two of the things listed are causing your baby to be unsettled in the evenings, or it may be a combination of them all. The important thing is to go through the list and tick off the possible reasons that you feel could be the cause of the problems you are having. Once you have your list of possible causes, using the advice in this chapter you can create a sleep plan to resolve each of the issues. Sometimes two or three issues can be resolved at once, or it may be that you have to resolve the problems in two or three different stages.

The main causes of unsettled evenings in babies aged one to six months are:

- Hunger
- Overtiredness
- Under tiredness
- Strong Moro (or startle) reflex
- Wrong sleep association

Hunger and the breast-fed baby

With any baby under six months I would always look at hunger as one of the main reasons why the baby was not settling well in the evening, particularly if the baby is 'cluster feeding' all evening.

Cluster feeding

Cluster feeding is a term used to describe a feeding pattern of young breast-fed babies who are very unsettled and need to feed constantly or very close together for a few hours at a time. Although it can happen at any time of the day, the most common time is between 6 and 10pm.

During the cluster-feeding period, the baby will often be very fretful, feeding for short spells before pulling off the breast and fussing or crying for several minutes before going back on the breast for several more minutes. As already mentioned, this pattern of feeding usually lasts between two and four hours before the baby eventually falls asleep. Often the baby will sleep for several hours after the cluster feeding, leading some mothers to believe that their baby is 'tanking up' during the cluster-feeding period, helping the baby sleep longer in the night.

Having had to resolve literally thousands of problems of cluster feeding or early-evening fussiness, I do not personally believe that the baby sleeps longer in the night because it has tanked up. I believe that the longer sleep in the night happens because, after nearly four hours of fussing and crying, the baby is simply exhausted and too tired to wake up. While a good weekly weight gain will indicate that a baby is receiving enough milk over a 24-hour period, it does not mean that he is getting enough milk at his bedtime feed in order to settle and sleep well in the evening. In nearly all the consultations where I have dealt with this type of early-evening unsettledness, the cause was low milk supply. This is a very common problem for breast-feeding mothers, especially later in the day. A low milk supply could be the reason why it may take these babies who are cluster feeding nearly four hours to get the same amount of milk as a baby who feeds well within an hour and then settles to sleep in the evening for three to four hours.

If you were to do an internet search on this problem you would find a huge amount of information claiming that this type of feeding behaviour in the early evening is totally normal and has nothing to do with low milk supply. In fact some authors go so far as to say that you should not supplement your babies at this time with a bottle of formula or expressed milk as it will decrease your milk supply. While I am in agreement that supplementing breast-feeds with formula or expressed milk *can* reduce a mother's milk supply, I would argue that this will not happen if the mother ensures that her breasts receive enough stimulation to prevent the milk supply reducing even further – by putting the baby to the breast often enough, in addition to expressing milk. I think that it is very sad that so many young babies are going through hours of distress every evening for weeks and often months because mothers are led to believe that offering a bottle of expressed milk once or twice a day when their milk supply is low is going to reduce their overall milk supply. The truth is that, if the problem is managed properly, it is possible to ensure that the baby receives a full feed in the evening so that he settles and sleeps well for several hours, while actually increasing the mother's milk supply at the same time.

Thousands of mothers have used my 'increased milk supply plan' (overleaf) and found that, within a week, they not only have a very happy, contented baby who is settling and sleeping well in the evening, but they have also increased the amount of milk that they produce in the evening. Very quickly they are therefore able to drop the supplemented bottle-feed and fully breast-feed their baby, knowing that their baby's feeding needs are now being fully met.

Increased milk supply plan

If your baby is under six months of age and not settling in the evening, it is possible the cause is a low milk supply. Following this seven-day plan will quickly help to increase your milk supply and solve the issue of your young baby not settling in the evening. The temporary introduction of top-up feeds will ensure that your baby is not subjected to hours of irritability and anxiety caused by hunger.

DAYS ONE TO THREE

6.45am	• Express 30ml (1oz) from each breast.
7am	• Baby should be awake and feeding no later than 7am, regardless of how often he fed in the night. • He should be offered up to 20–25 minutes on the fullest breast, then up to 10–15 minutes on the second breast. • Do not feed after 7.45am. He can stay awake for up to one to two hours, dependent on his age (see page 11).
8am	• It is very important that you have a good breakfast no later than 8am.

9am	• If your baby has not been settling well for his nap, offer him up to 5–10 minutes on the breast from which he last fed. • Try to have a short rest when the baby is sleeping.
10am	• **Baby must be fully awake now, regardless of how long he slept.** • He should be given up to 20–25 minutes from the breast he last fed on, while you drink a glass of water and have a small snack. • Express 60ml (2oz) from the second breast, then offer him up to 10–20 minutes on the same breast.
11.45am	• He should be given the 60ml (2oz) that you expressed to ensure that he does not wake up hungry during his midday nap. • It is very important that you have a good lunch and a rest before the next feed.
2pm	• **Baby should be awake and feeding no later than 2pm, regardless of how long he has slept.** • Give him up to 20–25 minutes from the breast he last fed on while you drink a glass of water. Express 60ml (2oz) from the second breast, and then offer up to 10–20 minutes on the same breast.

4pm	• Baby will need a short nap according to the routine appropriate for his age.
5pm	• **Baby should be fully awake and feeding no later than 5pm.** • Give up to 15–20 minutes from both breasts.
6.15pm	• Baby should be offered a top-up feed of expressed milk from the bottle. A baby under 3.6kg (8lb) in weight will probably settle with 60–90ml (2–3oz); bigger babies may need 120–150ml (4–5oz). (See box opposite for more on bottle-feeding quantities.) • Once your baby is settled, it is important that you have a good meal and a rest.
8pm	• Express as much as possible from both breasts.
10pm	• It is important that you express from both breasts at this time, as the amount you get will be a good indicator of how much milk you are producing. • Arrange for your partner or another family member to give the 10.30pm bottle-feed to the baby so you can have an early night.
10.30pm	• Baby should be awake and feeding no later than 10.30pm. He can be given a full feed of either formula or expressed milk from a bottle.

In the night	• A baby who has had a full feed from the bottle at 10.30pm should manage to get to 2–2.30am. He should then be offered 20–25 minutes from the first breast, then 10–15 minutes from the second.
	• In order to avoid a second waking in the night at 5am, it is very important that he feeds from both breasts.

Bottle-feeding quantities

To calculate how much milk a baby should be given when feeding from a bottle you need to know your baby's weight. Health authorities advise that babies under six months who are not on solids will need 70ml (2.5oz) for each pound of their body weight per day. So a baby weighing around 5.4kg (12lb) would need approximately 840ml (28oz) a day. You would then divide this by the number of feeds he is on per day to work out one feed. This is only a guideline; hungrier babies may need an extra ounce at some feeds. It is also important to understand that formula and breast milk are digested differently and that a breast-fed baby having breast milk from the bottle may need to feed sooner than a baby who is given formula from the bottle.

DAY FOUR

By day four, your breasts should be feeling fuller in the morning and the following alterations should be made to the above plan:

- If your baby is sleeping well between 9 and 9.45am, reduce the time on the breast at 9am to five minutes.
- The top-up at 11.45am can be reduced by 30ml (1oz) if he is sleeping well at lunchtime, or shows signs of not feeding so well at the 2pm feed.
- The expressing at the 2pm feed should be dropped, which should mean that your breasts are fuller by the 5pm feed.
- If you feel your breasts are fuller at 5pm, make sure he totally empties the first breast before putting

him on to the second breast. If he has not emptied the second breast before his bath, he should be offered it again after the bath, and before he is given a top-up.

- The 8pm expressing should be dropped and the 10pm expressing brought forward to 9.30pm. It is important that both breasts are completely emptied at the 9.30pm expressing.

DAY FIVE

- Dropping the 2pm and 8pm expressing on the fourth day should result in your breasts being much engorged on the morning of the fifth day; it is very important that the extra milk is totally emptied at the first feed in the morning.
- At the 7am feed the baby should be offered up to 20–25 minutes on the fullest breast, then up to 10–15 minutes on the second breast, after you have expressed. The amount you express will depend on the weight of your baby. It is important that you take just the right amount so that enough is left for your baby to get a full feed. If you managed to express a minimum of

120ml (4oz) for the 10.30pm feed, you should manage to express the following amounts:

(a) Baby weighing 3.6–4.5kg (8–10lb) – express 120ml (4oz)

(b) Baby weighing 4.5–5.4kg (10–12lb) – express 90ml (3oz)

(c) Baby weighing over 5.4kg (12lb) – express 60ml (2oz)

DAY SIX

By the sixth day, your milk supply should have increased enough for you to drop all top-up feeds, and follow the breast-feeding routines appropriate for your baby's age, as laid out in *The New Contented Little Baby Book*. It is very important that you also follow the guidelines for expressing set out in the routines. This will ensure that you will be able to satisfy your baby's increased appetite during his next growth spurt. Some mothers find it beneficial to continue with one bottle of either expressed or formula milk at the 10/10.30pm feed until your baby is weaned on to solids at six months as this will allow the feed to be given by your husband or partner, enabling you to get to bed earlier after you have expressed, which, in turn, will make it easier for you to cope with the middle-of-the-night feed.

Hunger and the bottle-fed baby

Hunger is not as common with bottle-fed babies as it is with breast-fed babies as you can see exactly how much the baby is getting at the feed and, in theory, if a baby is hungry the solution would be to just add more milk to the bottle and the problem would be resolved. To calculate how much milk your baby needs a day you need to multiply 70ml of milk for each pound of his body weight. Therefore if your baby weighs around 5.4kg (12lb) in weight he would need approximately 840ml (28oz) of milk a day, divided between the number of daily milk feeds he is having. If he is on five feeds a day, then he would need around 170ml (5½oz) a feed; if he is on six feeds a day, he would need around 140ml (4½oz) a feed.

When doing a split feed at 5pm and 6.15pm your baby will probably need more milk than he would if taking a single feed at 6.15pm. For example, if you have calculated that your baby needs 120ml (4oz) a feed, then when offering a split feed where there is a gap of around one and a half hours, you may find that he needs to take a total of 150–180ml (5–6oz) at the split feed. Experiment with how you split the feed; some babies need more at the 5pm feed and less at the 6.15pm feed, but if your baby is not settling at the 6.15pm feed, you should try giving less at the 5pm feed and more at the later split feed.

Aim to get your baby to take most of his daily milk requirement between 7am and 11pm. This way the middle of the night feed will gradually become later and later until your baby is sleeping through until the morning.

If your baby is not taking a full feed after his bath in the evening, he may fall asleep fairly quickly but then wake up an hour or so later out of genuine hunger. If he is very tired he may then only take a further couple of ounces before falling asleep again, only to wake up an hour or so later and repeat the same pattern of feeding.

One of the main causes of bottle-fed babies not taking enough milk at individual feeds is when the parents push their babies into strict four-hourly feeding schedules. Although formula-fed babies can normally go a little longer than breast-fed babies between feeds, if their feeding schedule is not in tune with their sleeping needs, it can result in them feeding too little when they are sleepy and then too much at the wrong times if they get over-hungry. This can then have an impact on the amount they drink at their bedtime feed in the evening. Too small a feed at this time when the baby is at his most tired will result in him having to feed two or possibly three times during the evening. I have known parents try to cajole their baby into taking more milk at the bedtime feed when he doesn't want it, leading to the baby getting very upset and the mother mistaking these cries for colic.

If your baby is taking too little milk at his bedtime feed, it is possible that the cause is too big a mid-afternoon feed, resulting in him taking less at the bedtime feed. Try reducing the 2.30pm feed by 30ml (1oz) to see if this encourages him to take more at the bedtime feed. If this doesn't resolve the problem, I would advise trying the following:

- Ensure he sleeps until 6 or 7am to stop him becoming overtired during the day.
- If he is taking too much milk during his afternoon feed, offer a split feed in the morning to increase

his earlier milk consumption so he is not so hungry at the afternoon feed. I recommend that the mid-afternoon feed should always be slightly less so that he would be encouraged to take a bigger feed at bedtime. I also recommend that the feed be given no later than 2.30pm.

- If your baby is too tired at bedtime to take a full feed, try offering a split feed at 5pm and 6.15pm.

Other causes of night wakings

If your baby fed well at 10.30pm and wakes earlier than 2am, the cause may not be hunger. The checklist below gives other issues which may be causing him to wake earlier:

- Kicking off the covers may be the cause of your baby waking earlier than 2am. A baby under six weeks who wakes up thrashing around may still need to be fully swaddled (see page 49 for how to swaddle). A baby over six weeks may benefit from being half-swaddled under the arms in a thin cotton sheet. With all babies, it is important to ensure that the top sheet is tucked in well, down the sides and at the bottom of the cot (for more on this, see page 47).

- The baby should be fully awake at the 10.30pm feed. With a baby who is waking up before 2am, it may be worthwhile keeping him awake longer, and offering him some more milk just before you settle him at around 11.15pm.

- If your baby is having a lot more sleep than the chart on page 11 suggests for a baby of his age, it is possible that the waking earlier in the night is being caused by too much daytime sleep. Obviously you can't just force your baby to suddenly stay awake longer during the day, but if you gradually increase your baby's awake time at one of the daytime slots by a minute or two every couple of days, this will increase his awake time without causing any distress.

- Your baby may be suffering from other discomfort, so do check the room temperature in case the room is too hot or too cold.

Overtiredness

Once you have made sure that your baby's feeding needs are being met properly in the evening, if he is still not settling the next thing to look at would be overtiredness.

Overtiredness is often a result of overstimulation. An overtired baby reaches a stage where he is unable to drift off to sleep naturally, and the more tired he becomes, the more he fights sleep. Babies from birth to around 12 weeks of age can usually stay awake happily for one to one and a half hours before getting tired. And from three months to around six months of age most babies will gradually start to stay awake a little longer at most of their waking slots, until they are awake for nearer two hours at a time. Therefore if your baby wakes up around 4.30/4.45pm from his late afternoon nap, he would need to be settled in his bed no later than two hours from the time he woke up, which would mean around 6.30/6.45pm.

It is important with babies under six months that they are not allowed to become overtired. A young baby who is allowed to become overtired, and stays awake for more than two hours, can become almost impossible to settle. Even if your baby sleeps until nearer 5pm for his later afternoon nap, it is possible that by the end of the day he is getting more tired and can't stay awake as long as he does at his earlier waking slots. If, despite getting the feeding right, your baby is still not settling well in the evening, I would aim to bring his bedtime routine forward for a short spell so that he is in bed by 6.30pm. Once your baby shows signs of taking longer to go to sleep at 6.30pm, you can gradually move the bedtime later until he is going into his bed at 7pm.

Signs of overtiredness

- He will get fussy and often turn his head to the side as if rooting for a feed
- He will start to yawn several times
- He may have bout of hiccups or sneezing
- He goes very quickly from fussing to inconsolable crying
- He arches his back and/or pulls up his legs up as if in pain
- Older babies tend to give more obvious signs, such as rubbing their eyes or pulling their ears

Dealing with overtiredness

Once overtiredness has set in it is important to calm your baby down before you attempt to settle him in his bed. If your baby is very young, try swaddling him securely (see page 49) so that he cannot wriggle around. Once swaddled, hold and shush him until he calms down. However make sure he doesn't get to sleepy on your shoulder or chest. If this happens you may find that soon after putting him in bed he may wake up because he misses the comfort of your chest. Some overtired babies will settle better if they are allowed some 'crying down' time; please refer to page 160 on how crying down works.

Sometimes an overtired baby who has calmed down will get a second wind and become very awake, so it is important not to try to settle him in his bed until he looks sleepy. It is better just to sit quietly with him until he does show signs of being sleepy before attempting to settle him.

With older babies who are too big to swaddle, holding them closely and firmly in a quiet room with some gently music will often help them calm down. And again, like the younger baby, it is always worth offering them a top up feed, to help get them calm and sleepy. Once your baby looks as if he is about to sleep, you should settle him in his cot and allow him a short spell of fussing or crying-down time. See also page 19 for further tips on breaking the cycle of overtiredness.

Undertiredness

Having ruled out hunger and overtiredness, the next thing that I would suggest you to look at is your baby's daytime sleep. Although not so common in very young babies, sometimes putting a baby down when he is not ready to sleep can cause him to not settle. Too much sleep after 3pm is often the cause of unsettled evenings, especially if your baby is over three months old and sleeping well at his morning nap and middle-of-the-day nap. If he is sleeping for more than 45 minutes at his late afternoon nap but not settling well at bedtime, try reducing the nap every day by five to ten minutes to see if he settles better in the evening. I have cared for lots of babies who, when sleeping well in the middle of the day, had to have their late afternoon nap restricted to no more than 15 to 20 minutes if they were to settle well in the evening.

For guidance on how long babies need to sleep during the day for the first six months, see the chart on page 11.

Strong Moro (or startle) reflex

During the first few weeks, the majority of babies have a very strong Moro reflex. This reflex is sometimes known as startle reflex because it usually occurs when a baby is startled by a loud sound or movement. The baby responds by throwing back his head, extending out his arms and legs, crying, then pulling his arms and legs back in. Even a baby's own cry can startle him to trigger this reflex. Also when laid down, the baby will sometimes suddenly start thrashing his arms and legs around. As the baby grows, this reflex gradually lessens and by five to six months it has disappeared altogether. I have observed many babies coming into a light sleep in the middle of the night and thrashing their legs up and down hysterically because they have kicked off their covers.

If your baby is under four months and not being tucked in securely with a sheet and blanket, then this could be a cause of him becoming unswaddled in the early part of the evening and waking several times. For this reason I believe it is very important that a baby is tucked in securely by his bed covers until the Moro reflex has totally disappeared; the sheet and blankets should be placed lengthways across the width of the cot and then two rolled hand towels pushed down between the spars and the mattress (see illustration below).

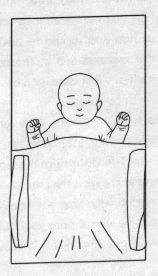

Parents will often say to me that their baby will sleep well from the late feed unswaddled and not tucked in, but I have found that they sleep so soundly after midnight because they are so exhausted from the disrupted sleep in the earlier part of the night, not because they are doing so naturally.

To eliminate the Moro reflex as a possible cause of your baby not settling well in the evening, please check my recommendations to help your baby feel more secure in his bed:

- Birth to six weeks: your baby should be fully swaddled with a non-stretch cotton sheet over the top of him and tucked in well under both sides of the mattress and at the bottom, so he cannot kick it off. (For details on how to swaddle, see the box opposite.)
- Six weeks to eight weeks: start semi-swaddling your baby at the late afternoon nap and then the morning nap. Then introduce the semi-swaddle in the evening and if he is sleeping well at the lunch time nap and finally, after the late feed.
- Eight to twelve weeks: once your baby is sleeping happily with one arm out of the swaddle at all

naps, gradually start introducing a half-swaddle in the same sequence as the semi-swaddle.

- Somewhere between four and six months your baby may start to roll onto his tummy. When this happens it is safest to remove all bedding from the cot and put your baby to sleep in a 100 per cent cotton lightweight sleeping bag. During the summer months I recommend a 0.5 tog sleeping bag or, in very hot weather, a muslin sleeping bag. Until he is capable of rolling from back to front and then from front to back, you will need to keep returning him to his back. (Please refer to page 109 for problems with transitioning from the swaddle to a sleeping bag and from your baby sleeping on his back to finding his own position in the cot.)

How to swaddle your baby

Full swaddle
1. Use a rectangular jersey cotton swaddling blanket. About 180 x 100cm is ideal. Place

your baby to the right of the centre of the blanket. Make sure the top of the blanket is slightly higher than the back of his neck.

2. Take your baby's left hand and point it outwards from his body.

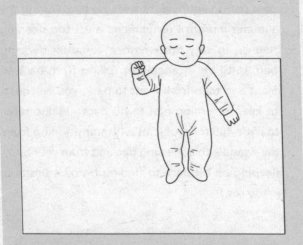

3. Draw the right-hand side of the blanket across his chest, then take the baby's left arm (encased in the blanket) and fold it over his chest, creating a fold in the blanket.

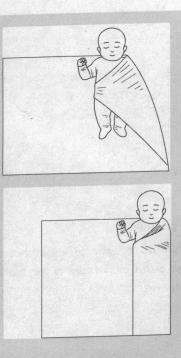

4. Gently tug it down so the blanket edge is sitting firmly around your baby's neck and tuck the excess blanket around his back and under his bottom.
5. Repeat the same procedure with baby's right hand.

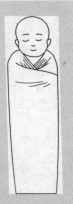

Semi-swaddle

Swaddle your baby as usual but leave the second arm free, wrapping the blanket under his left arm.

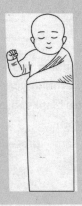

Half-swaddle

Swaddle your baby as usual but wrap the swaddle blanket under both arms instead of over his arms.

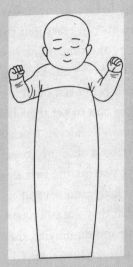

Always position your baby on his back with his feet almost touching the bottom of the cot so he cannot wriggle under the covers. For a video showing how to swaddle and half-swaddle, please go to: www.contentedbaby.com/video.htm

Sleep associations

As we have seen, one of the biggest challenges parents face in the early days is getting their baby to settle in the evening. It is taken for granted that it is normal for very young babies to be unsettled between 6 and 10pm. Parents are reassured that this is only a stage and that by the time a baby reaches 12 weeks he will be settling better in the evening. During this unsettled phase it is understandable that parents will do whatever they can to get their baby to sleep, and the evening usually results in much feeding, rocking or giving the baby a dummy to get them to sleep. Sadly, for many parents the first three months come and go very quickly and several months down the line they find that they are still having to spend hours feeding, rocking and dummying their baby to sleep.

If you constantly cuddle, rock, feed or use a dummy to get your baby to sleep, it is what he will come to associate with falling asleep. This does not often create a problem during the first few weeks, but once the baby's sleep cycles develop and he starts to come into a light sleep every 30–40 minutes a real problem can evolve. In my experience, babies who depend on their parents to help them get to sleep will, at around eight to twelve weeks, start to wake up increasingly in the night. Babies who were often feeding only once in the night end up feeding every couple of hours; others will not settle unless cuddled or rocked, or given the dummy.

During the very early days nearly all babies will fall asleep while feeding and usually they can be placed in the cot in a very sleepy state and stay asleep until the next feed is due. However, as they get older a baby may start to wake up 30–40 minutes after they have been put down in their cot. The parent assumes that the baby may not have fed well enough and will offer either a further breast-feed or a smaller bottle-feed. The baby may or may not return to sleep quickly. Sometimes they will need further assistance in the form of rocking or being given the dummy when they are put back in the cot.

If your baby is under eight weeks, this problem can be avoided by ensuring that you allow enough time to settle your baby at sleep times. Make a note of how long your baby can stay awake before he falls asleep then make sure that you allow a 10- or 15-minute wind-down period before he goes to sleep. If he has fed earlier and is unsettled but you are sure he is not hungry or windy, give him a cuddle or the dummy, but make sure that he is settled in his cot without the dummy before he falls asleep. If he has just had a feed and is falling asleep on the breast or bottle, try to rouse him slightly before you put him into the cot so that he is aware that he is going to bed. Provided he has been well fed and winded and is ready to sleep, he should drift off to sleep within five to ten minutes, although I have had a few babies who would fuss and fret for up to 20 minutes before settling off to sleep. Please see page 160 for tips on the 'crying down' method, which can be useful here.

If your baby is under eight weeks and is not settling well despite looking sleepy, it is important that you look closely at his feeding. In my experience the cause is usually one of three things: the baby is still hungry, the baby was too sleepy to take a big enough feed or he got sleepy during the feed and snuck in a little cat nap, which was just enough to give him a second wind.

If your baby is between birth and six months and you are confident that your baby's feeding has been sorted out, you are achieving the right balance of daytime sleep and any issues with bedding are resolved, then getting your baby to self-settle and sleep independently without the various sleep props should be the final thing you need to implement to get your baby totally self-settling and sleeping well in the evening until the late feed. However, before you attempt to remove the sleep props, I would strongly recommend that you follow the 'assisting-to-sleep routine' on page 157 for several nights. It will be much easier to remove the sleep props if your baby's body clock is used to sleeping at the same time every evening than if he is still being unsettled.

Through all my experience of working with children I have come to the conclusion that the key to ensuring good sleeping habits is to teach your baby to go to sleep in his basket or cot unassisted. Establishing the right sleep associations from an early age is vital if you wish to avoid long-term sleep problems.

In the very early days the majority of babies will fall asleep near the end of a feed, and they will be almost impossible to rouse. When placed in their bed, they will continue to sleep until the next feed. Somewhere between three and four weeks, when the baby starts to manage to stay awake for a slightly longer period, it is important that, particularly after his daytime feeds, he is put down before he gets into a deep sleep. If he does fall into a deep sleep near the end of the feed, try to rouse him a little before placing him in his bed, so that he is aware that he is going into it. Between two and three months the baby's sleep cycle changes and becomes much more apparent, with him coming into a light sleep 30 to 40 minutes after he has fallen asleep. If the baby gets into the habit of going into his bed in a deep sleep, when he comes into his light sleep he may not manage to settle back to sleep himself because he will be aware that he is in a different place from where he first fell asleep. If this is allowed to happen after every feed and at every sleep time, a pattern soon emerges where the baby needs repeated settling to sleep several times a night.

SIX TO TWELVE MONTHS

While the causes of unsettled evenings for older babies can often be the same as those of younger babies, how to deal with them can vary slightly, depending on the problem.

The main causes of unsettled evenings in babies aged 6 to 12 months are:
- Hunger
- Overtiredness
- Undertiredness
- Rolling over
- Wrong sleep association

Hunger and the breast-fed baby

At six months most babies have either been on solids for a short time or they have just started on solids. Many parents hope that the introduction of solids will see an end to unsettled evenings, and in many cases, if hunger is the only cause, then indeed some solids in the evening may help resolve the situation. However, a full milk feed is still essential at bedtime if a baby is to settle well in the evening. A baby of this age should be offered both breasts at the bedtime feed. If you find, however, that despite introducing solids and offering both breasts after the bath your baby is still unsettled, I think you have to consider that low milk supply in the evening could be the problem.

To rectify this, I would advise that, instead of offering both breasts after the bath, for a couple of nights you express as much as possible from both breasts at 5.30pm, after your baby has had solids at 5pm and is happy to play for a short spell. Bring the bath forward by 10 minutes to allow a bit longer for the milk feed. I would then first offer your baby a bottle with however much you have managed to express and then offer him both breasts. To avoid him getting too sleepy on the breast, I would alternate him back and forth between both breasts, offering five minutes at a time.

If he takes around 180ml (6oz) from the bottle and a feed from both breasts and is still unsettled in the evening, then I doubt the cause is really hunger. However, to totally eliminate the possibility I would recommend that in the morning you express a little milk that you can add to your evening bottle to make it up to a total of 240ml (8oz). Follow the same procedure as the previous night, but this time offer the full 240ml (8oz) feed. If he is still unsettled in the evening, then I think you can certainly rule out hunger as being the cause.

If your baby does settle well, then I would recommend that you continue to offer a bottle of expressed milk at this time, but follow the 'increased milk supply plan' on page 30 to increase your milk supply. Once you have increased your milk supply, you can go back to offering your baby a breast-feed in the evening, although you may have to continue to offer a small top-up bottle of expressed milk after he has had both breasts.

Hunger and the bottle-fed baby

Babies who reach six months and have started solids will still need a full milk feed at bedtime. A full milk feed for a baby of this age would normally be 210–240ml (7–8oz). If your baby is unsettled in the evening, or wakes up after an hour or so of being put down, and is taking a lot less than this, then low milk intake could be the cause.

The main reason why a baby of this age would not take a full milk feed is usually increasing solids too quickly at 5pm. Between six and seven months most babies will gradually increase their solid intake from one tablespoonful to six to eight tablespoonfuls. If your baby is eating a lot more than this, it would be advisable to reduce his solids so he is taking a full milk feed at bedtime.

Another cause of a baby not drinking enough milk at bedtime is because solids are being given too close to his milk feed. Try to allow at least one and a half hours between solids and his bedtime milk.

Finally, if your baby is getting very tired at bedtime and is falling asleep on the bottle, it would be advisable to bring his tea forward slightly to 4.45pm, so that you can then bring his milk feed forward a little so he is not too tired to take the full feed.

A typical day of a formula-fed baby would look something like the following:

7–7.30am   *Breakfast*
150–240ml (5–8oz) of milk.

4–6 teaspoons of dry oat cereal mixed with 60–90ml (2–3oz) of the milk with fruit *or* toast with fruit spread.

11.30am   *Lunch*

6 tablespoons chicken casserole *or* vegetable and lentil shepherd's pie *or* steamed fish with creamed vegetables.

Small drink of water from a beaker.

2.30pm   *Mid-afternoon*

120–210ml (4–7oz) of milk. If your baby is still having a small drink of milk prior to the lunch-time nap, offer less at this feed, so as not to reduce appetite for 5pm solids.

5pm   *Tea*

6 tablespoons vegetable bake *or* pasta with red pepper sauce. Cheese, rice cakes or yoghurt.

Small drink of water from a beaker.

6.30pm   210–240ml (7–8oz) of milk.

Some babies may still need a small late sleepy feed until they are seven to eight months.

Overtiredness

If you are confident that your baby is taking the right amount of solids and milk, but he is still unsettled in the evening, then overtiredness would be the next thing to consider. Most babies who are having a couple of hours' sleep in the middle of the day can get through happily to bedtime. However, if your baby is not sleeping well at the lunchtime nap and refuses to have a short nap in the late afternoon, it is possible that he is getting overtired at bedtime. To resolve this problem, first try pushing his morning nap slightly later and reducing it; this should help you push his lunchtime nap slightly later and hopefully he will also sleep longer, so that he can get through the afternoon without needing a late afternoon nap or becoming overtired. If this does not resolve the problem, then you may have to use the assist to sleep method to ensure your baby does have a short nap of 20 minutes in the late afternoon, so that he does not become overtired. If he refuses to do this, I would advise that you bring his tea and bedtime routine forward by 15 minutes so that he is not overtired at bedtime.

Undertiredness

Once babies reach six months most are down to two naps in the day. If they are having a nap in the morning, followed by a nap of a couple of hours at lunchtime, then they should not need a late afternoon nap. However, some babies continue to want to have a short nap in the late afternoon, even if they have slept well earlier in the day. If you find that your baby is still sleeping in the late afternoon despite having two good naps earlier in the day, I would recommend that you gradually reduce the late afternoon nap by a few minutes every couple of days until he can manage to get through to bedtime without it.

Rolling over

By the time your baby reaches six months he will have probably transitioned from a half-swaddle and a blanket to a lightweight sleeping bag. This time usually coincides with when a baby starts to roll over. Once your baby starts to roll over he may wake up crying in the evening when he comes into his light sleep because he has rolled onto his tummy and is unable to roll back onto his back. He may also have manoeuvred himself into the corner of the cot and got stuck. Until he is able to easily move himself around the cot and get himself out of difficult positions, you will have to quickly assist him back into a position that he is comfortable with. See Chapter 5 cot Gymnastics for how to deal with this problem.

Sleep associations

Having resolved any issues with feeding and sleeping, along with ensuring your baby is used to sleeping well in a sleeping bag, without any covers, the main cause of him being unsettled would be the wrong sleep associations.

Although the sleep associations for the older baby are the same as those for babies under six months – feeding and rocking to sleep, as well as using a dummy – dealing with them is *slightly* different, as the assisting-to-sleep method (page 157) that I recommend for younger babies rarely works with older babies. Older babies tend to fight sleep more and can become overtired or overstimulated if the assisting-to-sleep routine is implemented.

With an older baby who doesn't know how to go to sleep unassisted, eliminating the wrong sleep associations will be more difficult and some form of sleep training (see page 153) will probably be needed if unsettled evenings are to be resolved and a healthy sleeping pattern established. Establishing healthy sleeping habits also depends on several other factors: getting the feeding right and ensuring that your baby's physical, mental and emotional needs are being met also have a huge influence on how well he sleeps.

With the problems of feeding and rocking to sleep read on to Chapters 3 and 4.

3
Feeding to Sleep

In the early days nearly all babies will fall asleep while feeding, and as most can only stay awake for an hour or so at a time, and with feeds often taking up to an hour, it is easy to understand why they do so. Provided they have had a good feed, most babies will then sleep for a couple of hours before they are ready to feed again. At this stage feeding to sleep isn't really considered to be a problem. However, it becomes an issue once the baby starts to manage to stay awake for longer than an hour or so, which for some babies can be as early as three to four weeks. This usually coincides with a growth spurt where the baby needs to increase the amount of milk he drinks. If the baby is unable to settle to sleep without feeding, a pattern of feeding every couple of hours can quickly emerge. Therefore, instead of the baby increasing the amount he drinks at an individual feed, he is topped up with another milk feed when he needs to sleep, which results in a pattern of snacking. During the day this may not seem such a problem, but unfortunately most babies who get into the habit of feeding to sleep during the day will also expect the same during the night. While feeding to sleep is more common among breast-fed babies it can also become a habit with bottle-fed babies.

If you do a Google search for 'feeding to sleep' you will find thousands of articles on how it is normal for babies to feed to sleep during the first year, and also normal for them to wake and need to be fed several times a night during the first year. However, if you do another search for 'baby sleep associations' you will come across an equal number of articles telling you that the reason that your baby is waking up so much in the night is that he has learned the wrong sleep associations. What no one tells parents when they are encouraged to assist their baby to sleep by rocking or feeding, is just how hard it can be to break those habits once the baby becomes totally dependent on being assisted to sleep. When I worked personally with babies I always made sure that between the second and third week I got the baby going down sleepy but awake.

If your baby is over six weeks old, check out the lists below to determine whether he is at risk of learning the wrong sleep associations or whether he has already learnt them as a result of feeding to sleep:

Low risk of poor sleep associations

- After his first two morning feeds of the day and his mid-afternoon feed, your baby stays awake for an hour or longer and then will drift off to sleep without feeding.
- Your baby falls asleep while feeding after his bath, at the late feed or in the middle of the night, but then sleeps for more than three to four hours or until he is hungry.

Although the risk of a long-term sleep association is less likely with babies who are settling at some feeds, I would still recommend that you work on encouraging your baby to self-settle at the lunchtime nap and in the evening. The older your baby gets, the more defined his sleep cycles will become, so it is possible that he could go from sleeping longer spells at night to waking up and not settling back to sleep without a feed because he becomes more awake between his sleep cycles.

High risk of poor sleep associations

- Your baby is over six weeks old and needs to be fed to sleep at every daytime nap and rarely sleeps longer than 45 minutes at a time during the day.
- Your baby is over six weeks old and is still feeding two or three times in the evening and also between midnight and 7am.

With babies who are being fed to sleep at every sleep time, there is usually the additional problem of them having developed a habit of snacking instead of taking full feeds. This is something that has to be addressed properly when eliminating the feeding-to-sleep habit. It is very important that, if the baby is to self-settle, they have had a full feed, whether they are breast- or bottle-fed.

ONE-WEEK PLAN TO ELIMINATE FEEDING TO SLEEP

If your baby is under six months old, teaching him to self-settle without feeding will be much easier than for an older baby where the habit has become well established. Before starting this elimination plan I would recommend that you read Chapter 1 on understanding baby sleep rhythms and sleep associations. Having a good grasp of how feeding to sleep can affect your baby's ability to sleep well will help you understand the following plan for eliminating this habit.

In order for this plan to be successful, one of the first, most important steps, if you are not already doing so, is to adapt to a routine where your baby is fed upon waking, kept awake for a short spell and then settled to sleep (see *The New Contented Little Baby Book* for detailed, age-appropriate routines).

Under six months

Because your baby is used to being fed to sleep, it will also mean that he is used to feeding little and often, and will be genuinely hungry just prior to a sleep. Therefore, initially during the plan you will still need to feed him, otherwise it is very probable he will not settle to sleep at all and become overtired and very irritable. Bear in mind throughout the plan that babies under six months of age need to sleep again within a couple of hours of being awake.

DAYS ONE TO SEVEN

In order for the plan to work it is important that you wake your baby around 7am, regardless of when he last woke and fed in the night.

- Once you have woken your baby, feed him and keep him awake for up to two hours. If he shows signs of getting tired before the two hours, try topping and tailing him around that time, and then taking him to a different part of the house. I often find that a change of scenery is enough to help a baby stay awake a little longer.
- Offer him a top-up feed a good 15 to 20 minutes before you normally settle him to sleep for his morning nap. Do this feed in a bright room and do not allow him to fall asleep while feeding.

- Once he has had the normal length of time on the breast or the usual amount of milk from the bottle, you should then start to settle him to sleep for the morning nap.

- On the first day the aim is to get him to sleep by whatever means you can, other than feeding him. Start off by shushing and patting him in the cot (see page 155), but if you find that he hasn't settled within 20 minutes, if needs be, rock him to sleep. While it may seem that you are replacing one sleep association with another, this is only for a short period until he gets used to not feeding to sleep.

- Because he had his top-up feed earlier, you will probably find that he is hungry the minute he wakes, and it is fine to offer him a feed if he needs one. Even if he does not show signs of being very hungry, I would advise that you offer him a feed no later than 30 minutes after he woke. The aim here is to establish a pattern where he is taking most of his feed when he wakes up, instead of splitting it between a small feed when he wakes and a small feed when he is sleepy.

- Watching for signs of tiredness (see page 13), aim to offer your baby a top-up feed 15 to 20 minutes before he would normally settle for his lunch-time nap. If he is bottle-fed, offer him most of his top-up feed, but reserve 30ml (1oz) for settling him just prior to the nap. Ideally you want this second nap to be a longer nap. Therefore you can offer him a further short feed of no more than 5 minutes on the breast or the remaining 30ml (1oz) from the bottle. This time you can allow him to get more sleepy than at his earlier nap, but it is important that he isn't put in the cot fully asleep.

- If he wakes after 30 to 40 minutes, try to get him back to sleep whichever way you can, other than feeding him. If he doesn't settle back to sleep he will probably be ready for a catnap after his next feed. As this sleep will only be a short one, if possible it is better to take him out in the buggy to get him to sleep, rather than try to settle him in his cot.

- Depending on his age, if your baby is still having a late afternoon nap I would recommend that you again take him out in the buggy so that you do not have to worry about him settling without feeding in the cot.

- It is really important that your baby takes enough milk at the evening feed so that he sleeps three to four hours before he needs to be fed again. The problem is, because it is the end of the day, this is the feed that most babies get very sleepy on. Normally I would recommend that after the bath this feed is done in a quiet, dimly lit room. However, for the first three nights I would recommend that you instead offer your baby most of his bedtime feed as you would a daytime feed, in a bright room. You should then delay the bath slightly so that once he has had his bath, he only needs to feed for a short while before he will be ready to sleep.

- Again, as at previous sleep times, if need be rock, pat and shush your baby to get him to sleep.
- As you will probably already be doing the late feed and any middle-of-the-night feeds as sleepy feeds (a sleepy feed is where the baby is not woken properly to feed, just aroused enough to take the feed and then settled back in his cot, usually within 15–20 minutes) you can continue to do this.

You should follow the above plan for seven consecutive days, each day bringing the top-up feeds forward slightly by a few minutes until your baby has dropped the top-ups at his first feed of the day and after the mid-afternoon feed. You can continue to give a top-up feed prior to his lunchtime nap, and at the bedtime feed you can now go back to doing a split feed at 5 and 6.15pm, but ensuring that your baby is not fed to sleep.

The chart overleaf gives a visual insight on how the plan works during the first four days. Once your baby has got used to settling to sleep without feeding, you will have to address how to get him to totally self-settle without any assistance. How you do this will depend on how long it has been taking you to get your baby to sleep without feeding him. If you have managed to settle him within a few minutes with the minimum of rocking or shushing, then it should be fairly easy to resolve this by placing him in his cot sleepy but awake and gently stroking his forehead or patting his tummy for a few minutes until he drifts off to sleep. If you find that this actually makes him more upset, then it would be worth trying a few nights of 'crying down' to allow him to self-settle. Please refer to page 160 on how this works and to follow the crying-down method properly. If you are still spending quite a bit of time assisting him to sleep by rocking or patting, then I would suggest that your refer to page 157 and follow the plan on how to eliminate this.

	Routine while feeding to sleep	Day one	Day two	Day three	Day four
Night-time sleepy feed	4am: sleepy feed	4am: sleepy feed	4am: sleepy feed	4am: sleepy feed	4am: sleepy feed
Wake	7am: awake and feed	7am: awake and feed 8.30am: top-up feed	7am: awake and feed 8.15am: top-up feed	7am: awake and feed 8.00am: top-up feed	7am: awake and feed 7.45am: top-up feed
First nap	8.45am: fed to sleep	8.45am: in crib, shush-pat to sleep 9.20am: asleep	8.30am: in crib, shush-pat to sleep 9.00am: asleep	8.45am: in crib, shush-pat to sleep 9.00am: asleep	8.45am: in crib, shush-pat to sleep 9.00am: asleep
Awake	10am: awake and feed	10am: awake and feed 11.30am: top-up feed	10am: awake and feed 11.15am: top-up feed	10am: awake and feed 11.15am: top-up feed	10am: awake and feed 11.15am: top-up feed

Lunchtime nap	11.45am: fed to sleep	11.45am: in crib, shush-pat to sleep 12.15/12.30pm: asleep	11.30am: in crib, shush-pat to sleep 12/12.15pm: asleep	11.30am: in crib, shush-pat to sleep 12/12.15pm: asleep	11.45am: in crib, shush-pat to sleep 12.00pm: asleep
Awake	2pm: awake and feed	2.15pm: feed 4.00pm: top-up feed	2.15pm: awake and feed 3.45pm: top-up feed	2pm: awake and feed 3.30pm: top-up feed	2.15pm: awake and feed 3.00pm: top-up feed
Late afternoon nap	4.30pm: fed to sleep	4.30pm: in bed or pram, shush-pat or walk to sleep	4.30pm: in crib or pram, shush-pat or walk to sleep	4.30pm: in crib or pram, shush-pat or walk to sleep	4.30pm: in crib or pram, shush-pat or walk to sleep
Awake	5pm: awake and feed	5pm: awake and feed 6.15pm: top-up feed	5.00pm: awake and feed 6.15pm: top-up feed	5.00pm: awake and feed 6.15pm: top-up feed	5.00pm: awake and feed 6.15pm: top-up feed
Bedtime	6.30pm: fed to sleep	6.30pm: in bed, shush-pat to sleep	6.30pm: in crib, shush-pat	6.30pm: in crib, shush-pat	6.30pm: in crib, shush-pat
Night-time sleepy feed	10pm: sleepy feed	10pm: sleepy feed	10pm: sleepy feed	10pm: sleepy feed	10pm: sleepy feed

Six to twelve months

Once babies are weaned on to solids between six and seven months, the number of breast-feeds they need is normally reduced to around three to four feeds a day. Some breast-fed babies may still need to have a late feed or an early morning feed around 5 or 6am, but they should not be needing to feed two or three times in the night, or several times a day. However, if your baby is very dependent on feeds to get him to sleep, it is possible that the number of milk feeds he is having during the day is impacting on the amount of solids he is taking. Before you start to eliminate feeding your baby to sleep, it is important that you ensure that he is eating a reasonable amount of solid food, so that you can be confident the extra milk feeds are due to comfort and not genuine hunger.

Below is a guide of what a fully breast-fed baby of seven months would be eating and drinking (both breasts should be offered at each feed). If your baby's consumption of solids is a lot less than this, I would recommend that you look to increase his solids before you start the elimination plan.

5–7am	Breast-feed
7–8am	6–8 tablespoons of breakfast cereal and fruit
11.30am	6–8 tablespoons of chicken, fish or bean casserole
12.30pm	Breast-feed
2.30–3pm	Breast-feed
5pm	6–8 tablespoons of savoury pasta-type meal
6.30pm	Breast-feed
10pm	Breast-feed (optional, may be dropped in favour of feeding at 5am)

If your baby is feeding two or three times in the night, this will certainly be affecting his appetite for solids during the day, and in turn the low intake of solids during the day obviously means your baby will wake up looking for food in the night. This coupled with the fact that he needs to be fed to sleep during the day will probably mean that he is taking so much extra milk that he is not eating enough solids. To remedy this I would recommend the following:

- Because your baby is feeding in the night, you should count that as his breakfast milk and go straight into breakfast solids when he wakes. He can then be offered his usual top-up milk feed just prior to his morning nap, but as he will have hopefully eaten more solids than normal, this feed should be smaller.

- If you are offering him a breast-feed before and after his lunchtime solids, you should cut out the milk feed prior to the solids and that should encourage him to eat more solids. He can then be offered a top-up of milk prior to his lunchtime nap.

- I would recommend trying keep the middle of the afternoon a smaller feed, and offer him his teatime solids slightly earlier so that again he increases the amount that he takes.

Once you see an increase in his consumption of solids, you can then start the following plan below, confident that your baby's need for feeding to sleep is through habit and is not hunger-related.

DAYS ONE TO SEVEN

In order for the plan to work it is important that you wake your baby around 7am, regardless of when he last woke and fed in the night.

- If your baby has fed in the night, wake him up no later than 7am and go straight into solids, offering a small milk feed after he has had solids.

- Offer a top-up feed a good 15 to 20 minutes before you normally settle him to sleep for his morning nap. Do this feed in a bright room, and do not allow him to fall asleep while feeding.

- Once he has had the normal length of time on the breast or the usual amount of milk from the bottle, you should start to prepare him for his morning nap. With an older baby who is on a shorter morning nap, I recommend that the nap is done in the buggy so that you do not have to worry about him settling without feeding in the cot. I would also recommend that if your baby is having more than 30 minutes for his morning nap, you reduce it over a few days to 30 minutes or less until he is settling well at his lunch nap, which should be in the cot.

- Because he had his top-up feed earlier, you will probably find that he is hungry slightly earlier. If this is the case I would recommend that you bring his lunchtime solids forward slightly. If you have been offering him a milk feed before solids, I would advise that you go straight into solids, so that he is taking nearer the amount of solids recommended above. If he is fussy with solids, offer him as much as he will happily take, then wait around 20 to 30 minutes and then offer some more. Obviously do not force him to take more than he is willing, but try to increase the amount if he is taking much less than 6 tablespoons.

- Watching for signs of tiredness (see page 13), aim to offer him a top-up feed 15 to 20 minutes before he would normally settle for his lunchtime nap. Give him most of this feed in the living room, taking him to his room for the last five to ten minutes of the feed.

- If he gets very upset when you put him in the cot, you can pick him up and calm him down and, if needs be, assist him to sleep by rocking, patting or shushing. The main aim during the first couple of days is to get him to sleep whatever way you can, other than by feeding him.

- If he wakes after 30 to 40 minutes, try to get him back to sleep whichever way you can, other than feeding him. But if he has not gone back within 20 minutes I would just get him up and give him longer at his next nap.

Feeding to Sleep

- If he doesn't settle back to sleep he will probably need to have a short nap in the late afternoon. As this sleep will only be a short one, if possible it is better to take him out in the buggy to get him to sleep, rather than try to settle him in his cot. The length of this nap will depend on how long he slept at lunchtime. If it was less than an hour then you could allow between 45 minutes and one hour. If he slept between one and one and a half hours, then I would limit this nap to 20 minutes so that he is ready to sleep at 7pm. It is important that your baby does not sleep after 5pm if you want to make settling at bedtime easier.

- If your baby is used to a milk feed mid-afternoon and hasn't slept well at lunchtime, it is important that this feed be brought forward slightly, so that you do not risk him falling asleep on the breast. If he normally has his solids at 5pm, I would recommend that you do this afternoon feed no later than 3pm, so that his appetite is not affected for solids.

- If your baby is taking a lot less than six tablespoons of solids, and gets fussy after two to three tablespoons, I would recommend the same approach as at lunchtime: take him out of the high chair for 20 minutes or so and then try again.

- If you have split the solids, then you would need to delay the milk feed slightly, and instead of offering one full milk feed after the bath I would split the feed so that he is having most of it in the living room as opposed to his dimly lit bedroom, which is what I would normally advise at bedtime. I would recommend that you do this for the next three nights, and then delay the bath slightly so that once he has had his bath, he only needs to feed for a short while before he will be ready to sleep.

- A baby of this age who has been used to feeding to sleep for many months may possibly get very upset when not allowed to fall asleep on the breast or bottle. Therefore it may take a lot longer to settle him at this sleep and, as recommended for the lunchtime nap, if needs be rock, pat and shush him to get him to sleep.

- Any feeds after 7pm should be done as sleepy feeds, so you do not need to worry about him falling asleep while feeding. At this stage the main focus is on settling him to sleep during the day and in the evening without feeding.

The chart overleaf gives a visual insight on how the plan works during the first four days. Once your baby has got used to settling to sleep without feeding, you will have to address how to get him to totally self-settle without any assistance. How you do this will depend on how long it has been taking you to get your baby to sleep without feeding him. If you have managed to settle him within a few minutes with the minimum of rocking or shushing (see page 155), then is should be fairly easy to resolve this by placing him in his cot sleepy but awake and gently stroking his forehead or patting his tummy for a few minutes until he drifts off to sleep. If you find that this actually makes him more upset then it would be worth trying a few nights of 'crying down' to allow him to self-settle. Please refer to page 160 on how this works and to follow the crying-down method properly. If you are still spending quite a bit of time assisting him to sleep by rocking or patting, then I would suggest that your refer to page 157 and follow the plan on how to eliminate this.

	Routine of eight-month-old baby feeding to sleep	Day one	Day two	Day three	Day four
Night-time sleepy feed	3.00am: breast-feed or 150ml (5oz) formula	3.00am: breast-feed or 150ml (5oz) formula	4.45am: breast-feed or 180ml (6oz) formula	5.15am: breast-feed or 210ml (7oz) formula	5.30am: breast-feed or 210ml (7oz) formula
Awake	6.15am: awake 6.30am: breast-feed or 180ml (6oz) formula	6.15am: awake	6.45am: awake	6.50am: awake	6.45am: awake

Breakfast	7.30am: 2 tbsp of dry cereal mixed with milk and 2 tbsp of mashed fruit	6.30am: 4 tsps of dry cereal mixed with milk and 2 tbsp of mashed fruit 7.30am: breast-feed or 150ml (5oz) formula	7.00am: 6 tbsp of cereal with 2 tbsp of mashed fruit 8.00am: breast-feed or 90ml (3oz) formula	7.00am: 6 tbsp of cereal with 2 tbsp of mashed fruit 8.00am: breast-feed or 90ml (3oz) formula	7.00am: 6 tbsp of cereal with 2 tbsp of mashed fruit 8.00am: breast-feed or 120ml (4oz) formula
Milk feed and sleep	9.00am: breast-feed or 90ml (3oz) formula – feed to sleep	8.45am: breast-feed or 60ml (2oz) formula 9.15am: asleep	9.00am: breast-feed or 60ml (2oz) formula 9.15am: asleep	9.00am: breast-feed or 30ml (1oz) formula 9.30am: asleep	9.00am: breast-feed or 30ml (1oz) formula 9.30am: asleep
Awake	10.15am: awake	10.00am: awake	10.00am: awake	10.00am: awake	10.00am: awake
Lunch	11.30am: 3 tbsp chicken casserole – very fussy	11.00am: 5 tbsp chicken casserole – fed well	11.00am: 6 tbsp lamb hotpot – fed well	11.00am: 6 tbsp fish lyonnaise – fed well	11.00am: 7 tbsp spaghetti bolognaise – fed well

Milk feed and sleep	12.30pm: breast-feed or 180ml (6oz) formula – feed to sleep	12.15pm: breast-feed or 120ml (4oz) formula 12.30pm: asleep	12.15pm: breast-feed or 90ml (3½oz) formula 12.30pm: asleep	12.00pm: breast-feed or 90ml (3oz) formula 12.30pm: asleep	12.00pm: breast-feed or 90ml (3oz) formula 12.30pm: asleep
Awake and milk feed	2.45pm: awake 3.00pm: breast-feed or 210ml (7oz) formula	2.30pm: awake 2.45pm: breast-feed or 90ml (3oz) formula	2.30pm: awake 2.45pm: breast-feed or 90ml (3oz) formula	2.30pm: awake 2.45pm: breast-feed or 120ml (4oz) formula	2.30pm: awake 2.45pm: breast-feed or 120ml (4oz) formula

Tea	5.00pm: 2 tbsp pasta with 1 tbsp vegetables with tomato sauce	4.45pm: 4 tbsp vegetable root medley	4.45pm: 6 tbsp shepherd's pie	4.45pm: 6 tbsp corn chowder	5.00pm: 6 tbsp macaroni cheese
Milk and bedtime	6.00pm: breast-feed or 240ml (8oz) formula – feed to sleep	6.15pm: breast-feed or 240ml (8oz) formula 6.50pm: asleep	6.30pm: breast-feed or 240ml (8oz) formula 6.55pm: asleep	6.30pm: breast-feed or 240ml (8oz) formula 6.55pm: asleep	6.45pm: breast-feed or 240ml (8oz) formula 6.55pm: asleep
Night-time sleepy feed	10.00pm: breast-feed or 120ml (4oz) sleepy feed	11.45pm: breast-feed or 180ml (6oz) sleepy feed	11.45pm: breast-feed or 90/120ml (3/4oz) sleepy feed	11.45pm: breast-feed or 60/90ml (3/4oz) sleepy feed	11.45pm: breast-feed or 60ml (2oz) sleepy feed*

* Once the sleepy feed is down to 90ml (3oz) and your baby continues to sleep through for several nights this feed can be dropped.

Sometimes, with older babies, if the problem has gone on for quite some time, if the crying-down method is used he will actually cry up instead of cry down (see page 160). If you find that this is the case with your baby I would recommend that you shush and pat for a week, and then try again with the crying-down method. If it doesn't work the second time you may have to consider a tougher form of sleep training, such as controlled crying (see page 168). Controlled crying is something that should only be used as a last resort when all other methods are not working. Although it is not easy to implement controlled crying, it is worth remembering that good quality sleep is essential for your baby's health, both physical and mental, therefore you have to weigh up whether a few nights of more intense crying is worse in the long term for your baby than weeks and possibly months of disrupted sleep.

4

Rocking to Sleep

Rocking a baby is seen as one of the most natural things in the world to do with a baby. It is an instinctive response from parents when dealing with a baby who is well-fed but fractious or who is resisting sleep. In the early days, the rhythmic movement can usually, within a short space of time, calm the baby and he can then be placed in his cot asleep and happily stay there until his next feed is due. Indeed, rocking is so much encouraged that we have nursing chairs for parents who can sit and rock back and forth while feeding their babies, along with rocking cribs for babies to sleep in, swinging or bouncing chairs for babies to sit in and a whole range of other gadgets that are designed to move and that manufacturers promote as helping your baby sleep better.

Because babies have been used to constant movement for nine months while in the womb, it is natural that for most babies a short spell of rocking will quickly settle them. Of course, rocking is not the only movement that can calm and help induce sleep; there are many other forms of movement that will help settle a fractious baby. The following are just a few of some of the other methods of movement that parents use:

- Walking around with baby over the shoulder
- Standing up and swaying the baby back and forth
- Pushing the baby back and forth in the pram
- Putting the baby in an battery-operated baby swing
- Driving the baby around in the car until asleep

Using most of the above methods will usually get a very young baby off to sleep within 10 or 20 minutes. Most parents think that this small amount of time and effort is well worth it once their baby has settled and sleeps well until his next feed is due.

All of the above methods of assisting a baby to sleep rarely cause any problems in the first month, but usually somewhere between the first and second month the majority of these babies will very gradually start to need to be rocked slightly longer and longer before they can get themselves off to sleep. It is such a gradual thing that most parents do not even notice initially that they are spending longer getting their baby to sleep, of if they do they assume that as the baby gets older that he will start to learn to self-settle himself to sleep and need less rocking. Certainly I am sure that with some babies that this does happen, and the parents one day just place the baby in his cot without rocking and he happily drifts off to sleep. However, for the majority of babies this simply does not happen, and parents find themselves months down the line spending anywhere between 20 minutes to an hour or more getting their baby off to sleep for naps and in the evening.

As the baby nears six months and his sleep cycles are really well-established, parents will end up in a situation where the baby will sleep no longer than 30 or 40 minutes in the day, then wake up and need to be rocked back to sleep, and in this pattern can continue well into the night with the baby becoming awake every couple of hours needing to be rocked back to sleep.

If you find that your baby is starting to become more difficult to settle at sleep times and waking up more in the night, but not looking for a feed, then weaning him off being rocked is essential if you want him to sleep for longer at nap times and sleep consistently through the night. Fortunately, weaning a baby off being rocked to sleep is easier than weaning a baby off being fed to sleep.

ELIMINATING ROCKING TO SLEEP

Before you start to wean your baby off being rocked to sleep, I would suggest that you check out the daily sleep requirement chart on page 10. While the sleep needs of individual babies do differ, it will give you an idea of how long your baby should be sleeping for his age. If he is sleeping much more than the recommended amount of time, I would suggest that before you start the plan that you gradually reduce the amount of daytime sleep he is having, until it is nearer the amount recommended in the chart for his age.

Preparation stage: adjusting the daytime sleep

In my experience, the reason that a lot of babies start to take longer to settle in the evening is that parents do not start to cut down their babies' daytime sleep as they get older. As a baby grows, he will start to need less sleep over a 24-hour period, and there is no guarantee that he will automatically reduce his daytime sleep. When this is the case, he will often start to cut down on his night-time sleep. The first sign of this is when the baby starts to take longer to settle in the evening. He then needs more and more rocking to get him to sleep, and a vicious cycle emerges where he needs more sleep during the day because he has lost sleep at night.

Obviously you can't suddenly just reduce his daily sleep by an hour or so all at once. But by following the three simple steps below, you should fairly quickly have reduced your baby's daytime sleep to the amount recommended for his age:

- Gradually push his first nap of the day later by five minutes every few days, and reduce it by five minutes or so until he is sleeping for the amount I advise in the morning for a baby of his age.

- At the same time as pushing the morning nap later and reducing it, you should be able to push his next nap on later and nearer to the times I recommend. Ideally the second nap of the day should come somewhere between 12 noon and 1pm, depending on your baby's age. If your baby has been having a shorter nap in the middle of the day and still needing a late afternoon nap, following these steps should help him to sleep longer for the mid-day nap. With babies under six months, they normally need a nap of between two to two and half hours. Between six months and one year, this normally reduces to around two hours.

- Once the mid-nap is taking place at the right time for his age, you should then be able to either reduce the late afternoon nap, or even cut it out altogether if he is nearer six months or older.

This preparation time spent getting your baby's daytime sleep times right will go a long way to ensuring that he is really ready to sleep at bedtime and make eliminating the rocking to sleep much easier.

During this preparation stage, it is fine to still assist your baby to sleep but you should follow these guidelines:

- You can pat and shush him in your arms until he falls asleep (see page 155), but all other movement should be avoided. Do not walk him around the room or sway him from side to side in your arms.
- Once your baby is very sleepy, it is important that you should very gently move him from your shoulder or your chest into the crook of your arms.
- If he starts to stir, quickly and gently grasp his two arms across his chest with one hand, so that he does not thrash around and wake up. Once you feel him going into a deeper sleep again, you can then release his arms but keep your hand firmly on his chest.
- Once you have reached a stage where you feel he is in a deep enough sleep to put in his cot, you can then gently lower him into the cot, but continue to hold your hand firmly but gently on

his chest until you are confident that he is in a deep sleep.

Once you are confident that your baby is having the correct amount of sleep for his age and is settling to sleep with only being held and not rocked, you can then move on to stage two of the plan.

Stage two: one week to fully eliminate rocking

DAYS ONE TO THREE

- Always start the second stage of the plan in the evening when your baby is at his most tired.
- Use the method above, using patting and shushing to get your baby to a sleepy stage, but do not get him quite as sleepy as he was during the preparation stage.
- Each night reduce the time he is on your shoulder or across your chest, and increase the time he is in the crook of your arm with your hand on his chest.
- Start to put him in the cot sleepy but awake and remain by the side of the cot with either your hand on his chest or holding his hands across his chest.

- If you sense that he is about to become unsettled and more awake, you can gently roll him onto his side and shush and pat him until he falls asleep. If he is under six months it is important that once he is asleep that you make sure that he is lying on his back. Putting him on his side should only be done during the shushing and patting stage of getting him to sleep. With an older baby of six months or more, I find it better to move him onto his tummy and hold down with one hand and shush and pat with the other. (See page 155 for more on the shush and pat technique.)

- The aim during the first three nights is to get your baby used to falling asleep in his cot, not to totally self-settle at this stage.

- During the day the same method should be used to settle your baby for naps.

DAY FOUR

- On the fourth day you can still use the above method to settle your baby for his naps, but in the evening you should allow him to self-settle using the crying-down method as described on page 160.

- If you find that after ten minutes your baby is crying up instead of crying down (see page 160), you can help calm him down by shushing and patting him, but this should only be done until he calms down; he should not be shush-patted into a deep sleep.

- You can return to the room every ten minutes and shush-pat him to calm him down, but it is important that you do not shush-pat him to sleep.

DAY FIVE

- On the fifth day you should start to settle your baby in his cot and use the crying-down method, checking him after ten minutes if he is crying up and, if needs be, shush-patting him to calm him down.

- It is really important that if you have to shush and pat him that you do not shush-pat him into a deep sleep.

- During the days of self-settling, it may take him longer to get to sleep and he will, in effect, lose some sleep. It is important that he does not become overtired, but it is also important that you do not allow him to sleep much longer past his wake-up time. Allowing a baby to sleep too much past his usual wake-up time could affect his feeding and put the rest of his day out, so this should be avoided. I find it best to make a compromise; for example, if he took 20 minutes longer to go to sleep, I would allow him to sleep 10 minutes past his usual wake-up time.

DAY SIX

- By day six your baby should be starting to self-settle within ten to twenty minutes of crying down. If not, I would recommend that you gradually increase the time you allow him to cry down by a further five to ten minutes.

- If you have reached a stage where your baby is going in his cot sleepy but awake and settling with the minimum of shush-patting, he is almost there in terms of self-settling. Therefore, it is important that, if needs be, you allow him longer to cry down. Increase the crying-down time to around 20 minutes. If he is crying up after 20 minutes you can go in and reassure him very quickly by standing by the cot and saying 'shush, shush' but not actually touching him.

- This can be repeated every 15 to 20 minutes until he has settled himself to sleep.

DAY SEVEN

- By the seventh day you should have reached a stage where your baby is self-settling within five to ten minutes, although some babies who fight sleep may take a little longer. The important thing to remember is that for the last week he has not been falling asleep in your arms but in the cot. It is important to not to backtrack at this stage and revert to assisting him to sleep in your arms.
- If you find that he is crying up after 20 minutes instead of crying down, then I would recommend that you go back to the day five plan and follow it for a few more days before moving on to days six and seven.

5

Cot Gymnastics

At around four to six months the majority of babies start moving around in the cot and usually rolling onto their sides or their tummies. Some will adapt to sleeping well on their tummies, and others will get very upset if they roll onto their tummy and have not yet learned how to roll over onto their back again. Between nine and twelve months babies usually start to sit or stand up in the cot. Again, if a baby has not learned how to lie down from a sitting position or to get down from a standing position in the cot, he will get upset and sleeping can become very disrupted. In this chapter I will deal with the different challenges that each sleeping transition makes and how to quickly resolve the night wakings that often accompany them.

SWADDLING YOUR BABY

When I first started working with babies over 30 years ago it was normal practice to fully swaddle babies and place them on their side, with a rolled up towel at their back and their front to keep them in place. In addition they would then be tucked in securely with a sheet and one or two blankets, depending on the temperature. It was quite common in those days to swaddle for three to four months, and often longer. Once the babies were unswaddled, they would then be placed on their tummy to sleep, but still tucked in securely for many months, and some parents would continue this tucking in until their babies were a year old.

Since those days there have been a lot of changes in the advice on the best sleep positions for babies and the most widely recognised recommendation is to always place your baby on his back to sleep (unless your doctor has advised you of a medical reason to do otherwise). Since the 'back to sleep' campaign, there has been a big reduction in the number of babies who die from sudden infant death syndrome (SIDS). The Lullaby Trust recommends that it is important that you place your baby on his back for *every* sleep, as the chance of SIDS is particularly high for babies who are sometimes placed on their front or side. It also recommends that if your baby has rolled onto his tummy, you should turn him onto his back again. Although the research into SIDS is still ongoing, all experts agree that laying babies on their backs to sleep is the safest position until they reach an age where they are strong enough to push themselves up with their arms and can roll from back to front and back again. Once they reach this stage, parents are advised that they no longer need to keep repositioning their baby onto his back if he rolls onto his tummy; instead they can leave him to find the sleep position that he finds most comfortable.

The best way to make sure your baby sleeps on his back is to do this from day one and keep putting him to sleep on his back for every day and night-time sleep. If you have any concerns about how your baby sleeps, please speak to your health visitor or GP.

During the first year there are several different transitions of how babies will sleep in their beds.

In the first few weeks after birth, the majority of parents I have worked with swaddle their baby, often using one of the many specially designed swaddle blankets available on the market. Somewhere between the second and fourth months, the baby will be transferred from being fully swaddled to half-swaddled, and possibly still being tucked in. Then finally, around six months, he will go from being half-swaddled to a 100 per cent cotton lightweight sleeping bag.

Without a doubt, the majority of newborn babies sleep much better when swaddled, and for that reason many parents continue to swaddle their babies for many weeks and often months. When they eventually attempt to put their baby to sleep unswaddled he often refuses to settle and, when he eventually does, will wake up several times a night crying. This is particularly true of babies who have a very strong Moro reflex (see page 46 for more on this). Because the Moro reflex can be very strong in some babies until they are six months or older, I know that it can be a real struggle for some parents getting their baby to sleep on his back, particularly once the baby goes from being fully swaddled to unswaddled. While I am a great believer in swaddling very young babies, as I think it does help establish a good sleep pattern, continuing with a swaddle so an older baby sleeps longer in the night is not something I would recommend. Overheating is believed to be another contributing factor in SIDS and for that reason I advise that parents start to get their babies used to sleeping unswaddled from around six weeks, even if it means a slight backtrack on the length of time that they sleep in the night. Swaddling, like the dummy, can become a sleep prop, and if allowed for too long can actually end up causing a sleeping problem instead of helping the baby sleep better.

From swaddle to sleeping bag

If your baby is over two months and has become dependent on the swaddle to sleep, and you find that he has started waking up more in the night when you attempt to unswaddle him, the stages outlined overleaf will gradually get him used to not being fully swaddled and help to prepare him for sleeping soundly without a swaddle.

Stage 1	Semi-swaddle (one arm in and one arm out – see page 52 for an illustration) your baby for his morning and late afternoon naps. Alternate arms at each sleep time. Continue to fully swaddle at the lunchtime or longest nap of the day, and during the night.
Stage 2	Once your baby is used to sleeping with one arm out at the morning and late afternoon naps (this usually takes one or two days), you should then start to half-swaddle (under the arms – see illustration on page 53) at these naps. You should also then start to semi-swaddle during the lunchtime nap and during the first part of the evening.
Stage 3	Once your baby is used to the semi-swaddle at the lunchtime nap and during the first part of the evening, you can then start to semi-swaddle from the late feed.

I recommend that you allow a week for this preparation before moving on to the one-week plan opposite.

One-week plan for removing the swaddle

Your baby should now be half-swaddled at the morning and late afternoon naps and semi-swaddled during the lunchtime nap and at night. Once you reach this stage you are ready to either half-swaddle your baby or put him in a sleeping bag during the lunchtime nap and at night. Following the plan below, within a week your baby should be sleeping happily either half-swaddled or in a sleeping bag for at all his sleep times.

DAYS ONE TO THREE

Continue to semi-swaddle your baby for his longest nap of the day. I find that it is best to introduce the half-swaddle in the evening as that is when he will be at his most tired and less resistant to fighting sleep.

In the evening settle your baby in his cot half-swaddled or in a sleeping bag. Ensure that he is in the 'feet to foot' position (with his feet at the end of the cot) and that the top sheet is tucked in well under the mattress. I would recommend that you put the sheet lengthways across the width of the cot so that there is a least 30cm (12in) tucked in under the mattress at the far side of the cot and you are able to tuck in at least 20cm (8in) under the mattress at the side you put your baby down. This way it is impossible for your baby to kick the covers off. There is no need for blankets, only one thin cotton flat sheet across the baby to ensure that he is securely tucked in. If you decide to replace the half swaddle with a sleeping bag, it is important that you choose one that is a 0.5 tog [or in hot weather a muslin one,] so there is no risk of the baby over-heating. I would still use a thin sheet across the cot to ensure that the baby is not thrashing around. Please refer to page 47 on how to tuck the baby covers well in the cot.

If your baby still has a fairly strong Moro reflex, you may wish to stay near the cot for the first couple of nights when you settle him. If you find that he is resisting sleep and thrashing his arms up and down, I would recommend that you stand over the cot and gently hold his hands over his chest to help him drift off to sleep. Once he has gone to sleep I would recommend that you still stay near the cot so that when he comes into a light sleep you can quickly hold his hands again across his chest until he drifts back into a deep sleep again. Once he is in a deep sleep, let go of one arm and once he is completely relaxed let go of his other arm. In my experience, if you can help your baby through his first light sleep phase of the evening, he usually manage to settle himself back when he comes into the next light sleep stages.

After the late feed and middle-of-the-night feeds, if you are still doing them, you may find that you have to follow the same procedure.

DAYS FOUR TO SIX

If your baby is not already self-settling by the fourth night I would recommend that you now allow him a short period to see if he will settle himself. Obviously you do not want him working himself up into a state, but I would certainly leave him for five to ten minutes to see if he can get himself off to sleep. If he is crying I would suggest that you gently hold one of his arms, but preferably not both. You will need to carry out this self-settling procedure when you put him down after night feeds as well. In my experience, by this stage the majority of babies are self-settling within a very short time.

DAY SEVEN

I deliberately leave the lunchtime nap until the very end of the unswaddling process; the reason being that if the lunchtime nap goes wrong it can result in a very overtired baby, making the evening settling to sleep more difficult. Once your baby is self-settling and sleeping unswaddled at night, you can then unswaddle him at the lunchtime nap, confident in the knowledge that he can settle himself back to sleep when he comes into a light sleep.

The baby goes from being fully swaddled to semi-swaddled to half swaddled or being put in a sleeping bag, until he is tucked in with a thin flat cotton sheet that goes well under the mattress to stop him kicking it off. This will help him avoid thrashing his legs up and down when he comes into a light sleep and waking himself up fully. Once a baby starts to roll back and forth, the sheet would be removed and he would be in a sleeping bag.

ROLLING OVER

Between the ages of six and nine months the majority of babies start to roll from their back to their front, although some babies may do so much earlier. Until your baby can safely roll from back to front and then from his front to his back again, you will need to help him if he wakes in the night distressed because he can't get himself from his tummy to his back. Once your baby starts rolling over and moving around the cot it is essential that you remove all sheets and blankets and put him to sleep in just a sleeping bag, to avoid the risk of him getting tangled up in the bedding and suffocating. The current guidelines from The Lullaby Trust is that soft toys and comforters should not be placed in the cot with a sleeping baby until he is at least 12 months old. According to the American Academy of Paediatrics, pillow-like toys, blankets, quilts, cot bumpers and other bedding increase the risk of sudden infant death syndrome (SIDS) and death by suffocation or strangulation.

The majority of babies usually learn at around six to nine months how to roll from back to front and front to back. However, until that happens it can often mean several wakings a night where you have to reposition your baby back onto his back. It could also lead to a long-term habit where a baby capable of rolling will not do so, because he associates or gets used to his parents doing it for him in the night. For these reasons, I suggest encouraging your baby to practise rolling from back to front and front to back during the day, which I believe can speed up the rolling process.

Since it was recommended that babies sleep on their backs, there is a lot of emphasis of encouraging lots of daytime tummy time with babies, so they develop strong neck and arm muscles. However, it is equally as important that babies are encouraged to spend lots of time playing on their back and both sides as well as their tummy, so that they develop the good movement they need if they are to quickly learn to roll from back to front and then back again. Keep time in baby swings and bouncer chairs to a minimum.

You can encourage your baby to play on his side using the aid of toys and books. Initially, he may need your help staying on his side by supporting him from the back. Once he is happy laying on his side playing with his toys, gradually move them just out of his reach, and his natural instinct will be to cross his top leg over to help him reach the toy, which will be the start of him learning how to roll from his side to his tummy.

Once your baby has become confident about rolling back and forth from his tummy to his back, it is advisable not to rush to him the minute he cries out. Allow him a short spell to settle himself; otherwise he will become dependent on you to help him get back to sleep.

SITTING UP

Once your baby has learned how to sit up and get from the sitting-up position to laying on his tummy while playing, he should be put in the cot in the sitting-up position and encouraged to lie himself down.

STANDING UP

Between seven and nine months many babies will start pulling themselves up in the cot, but will not be able to get themselves back down to the sleeping position. Again, they will need some help getting back down until they have learned to do it themselves.

I have read lots of advice in parenting forums suggesting that by leaving the baby to cry for a few nights he will quickly learn how to get himself back down from the standing position. This is not something that I would recommend as I know of several babies who were left alone crying, which resulted in them stumbling and falling over in the cot, banging their heads on the wooden spars. This only resulted in them being frightened of being put in their cots and therefore standing up even more in an attempt to get out.

As with rolling over, a long-term habit can set in if you do not teach your baby how to get himself back down. Once your baby has learned how to pull himself up in the cot, you should spend several times a day teaching him how to lower himself from the standing position in the cot. You can do this first of all by helping him to practise lowering himself on the outside of the cot. Stand him up facing the spars of the cot and put his hands around them. Kneeling behind him and holding your hands over his, teach him to bring his hands down the spars of the cot as he lowers himself. If he is unsure how to bend his legs while he is doing this, you can try holding only one of his hands, while gently pushing his legs into a bending position. If you do it often enough, within a few days he will start to get the hang of it.

At this point you should start to put him in the cot standing up at sleep times and encourage him to lie himself down: kneel down next to the cot and hold his hands with yours around the bars of the cot, then encourage him to lower himself down to the mattress. It is important that you kneel on the floor while doing this – your face will then be lower than his at the starting point so he will be more keen to get down to your level. Once he has got from the standing position to the sitting position, it is important that you then encourage him to go from the sitting position to the sleep position of his choice.

Once he has learned how to get himself down, it is important that you physically reduce the amount of help you give him in the night, instead encouraging him to lie down himself, saying to him 'down you go', or words to that effect.

6

Dummy Addiction

When I worked with parents in their homes, the majority of the babies I helped care for were given a dummy in the first few months. If used with discretion, I find the dummy to be a great asset, especially with a 'sucky' baby or one who gets fussy and irritable prior to sleep times. However, my advice has always been that the dummy should be used to calm a tired or irritable baby and, if necessary, help settle him at sleep times, but it should always be removed before he actually falls asleep. In my experience, allowing a baby to fall asleep with a dummy in his mouth is one of the worst sleep association problems to try to resolve; if a baby becomes 'addicted' to the dummy he will wake up several times a night and be unable to get back to sleep unless given the dummy.

Some recent research has suggested that using a dummy when putting your baby down to sleep may reduce chances of Sudden Infant Death Syndrome (SIDS). The Lullaby Trust advises that if you use a dummy, it is very important that you should ensure that you wait until breast-feeding is established first (about a month), and make sure you offer it for *every* sleep. This advice is echoed by The UNICEF UK Baby Friendly Initiative; it says that research shows dummies may be protective but that infants may be 'at greater risk of SIDS if they routinely use a dummy but have not been given their dummy on a particular night.'

The Lullaby Trust offers some key points for anyone who chooses to use a dummy for putting their baby to sleep: 'Don't force your baby to take a dummy or put it back in if your baby spits it out. Don't use a neck cord. Don't put anything sweet on the dummy, and don't offer it during awake time.' There are also certain health concerns to be aware of. The UNICEF UK Baby Friendly Initiative warns about potential risks of dummy use, which include increased risk of ear infection and dental problems, as well as 'risk of accidents such as obstruction of the airway'. If you have any safety concerns about the use of a dummy, I would urge you to contact

The Lullaby Trust directly to discuss the matter with them personally.

Since the publication of the advice that babies should be put to sleep at every sleep with a dummy, I have seen a huge increase in sleeping problems where the baby's reliance on the dummy has become so bad that parents can find themselves replacing it every 30 to 40 minutes from early evening right through to 6 or 7am. I have witnessed first-hand the serious affect that the lack of sleep has both on the baby and parents when this happens.

If this is the case for you, please see below for some practical strategies to help you cope with the lack of sleep that can come with the persistent use of the dummy.

SURVIVING DUMMY ADDICTION

The Lullaby Trust recommends that you withdraw the dummy from your baby between six and twelve months old. Until your baby reaches an age when you feel comfortable getting rid of the dummy completely, I would recommend that you give up on battling bedtime out if your baby is just not settling in the evening without it. One of the things that most parents find really difficult to cope with when their baby is dependent on the dummy is constantly trying to settle their baby in the evening when he wakes every 30 to 40 minutes needing the dummy. Sometimes a baby wakes up after 30 to 40 minutes looking for the dummy, but even when given the dummy he can take a further 30 to 40 minutes to return to sleep, only to wake up again and the same pattern repeats itself.

If this is what is happening with your baby in the evening, I would recommend that you don't even attempt to settle your baby for a longer sleep around 6 or 7pm. Instead, until you are in a position where you can implement a plan to totally eliminate the dummy, I would advise that for a short period you aim to settle your baby for a nap and then extend his day by having a further one or two awake periods during the evening, so that he is not getting himself worked up into a fretful state looking for the dummy.

For this method to work you will need to adjust your baby's feeds so that when he wakes he can have a small feed and then stay awake happily. How long he will stay awake for will depend on his age:

babies under three months will probably manage to stay awake between one to two hours, and babies between three and six months usually manage to stay awake for up to two hours.

THE EXTENDED-DAY METHOD

- If your baby's bedtime is normally around 7pm, I would recommend that you give him a small milk feed at 5pm, then, instead of starting his bath and bedtime routine at 6.15pm, that you just feed him, then settle him for a nap.
- Hopefully, he will sleep for somewhere between 45 minutes to one and a half hours. As he had a small feed within the last couple of hours, he will probably not be very hungry when he wakes, but if he is very irritable offer him a small top-up feed so that he can stay awake happily. This will be for around one to two hours depending on his age.
- Treat this awake time like you would his other daytime awake slots. However, if he is irritable you may find that he prefers to just be cuddled on your lap, rather than play. This is absolutely fine.

Remember, what you are trying to achieve here is to have him awake slightly more in the evening, so that he is not needing to be given the dummy repeatedly to get him back to what is probably a very disrupted sleep.

- Depending on his age he will be tired again after one to two hours of being awake, and you should aim to give him another short nap before his bath and bedtime routine.

- Usually the bath and bedtime routine comes between 5 and 7pm. However, using the extended-day method, your baby's bath and bedtime routine will now come somewhere between 9 and 10.30pm, depending on when he last woke.

- For example, if he woke up from his last nap at 9pm, you would probably start his bath around 9.30pm, so that he is feeding around 10pm and settled in his bed around 10.30pm. Depending on when he fed, he may need a split feed at 9pm and 10pm.

- Please refer to the chart below on how to adapt and adjust the feeding and sleeping early evening, so that your baby still takes a really good late feed.

5pm	Tea time solids as usual
5.45pm	Offer his milk earlier so that he takes less now and more at 10.30pm
6.30pm	Settle baby for a nap – this can be in his pram or as you take him for a walk in his buggy
8.30/9pm	Wake baby up and have some social time before his bath
9.00pm	Offer him a small milk feed if he seems hungry
9.30pm	Start bath and bedtime routine
10.00pm	Bedtime milk feed and wind-down time done in his room

Obviously, your baby may still wake up in the night for the dummy, but you should find that because he has been awake more in the evening, the wakings in the night are slightly less. It is also important to remember that the aim of this plan is to reduce the stress in the early evening of constantly trying to get a fretful baby who is waking up several times needing the dummy to sleep. The above method will not resolve his need for the dummy, but it should make things a little easier until your baby has reached an age where you feel comfortable about tackling the dummy dependency problem.

DITCHING THE DUMMY

Once you have decided the time is right to tackle your baby's dummy dependency problem, you will have to decide whether to totally eliminate the dummy or allow your baby to have it at selective times during the day – when he is bored or tired, for example. In my experience, I find that parents who do not totally eliminate the dummy altogether can all too often end up offering it to their baby again at sleep times. Therefore, my opinion is that if you are going to eliminate it at sleep times it will be easier in the long term to eliminate it totally and not have a dummy in the house at all. You will not then be tempted to resort to it a few weeks down the line.

There is a lot of advice about how to ditch the dummy, many claiming to be 'gentle', promising a method that involves 'no crying'. One of these such methods involves allowing the baby to suck on the dummy and, as the baby's sucking lessens just prior to him falling asleep, you remove the dummy. While I am sure that this method works for some babies, it does not work for the majority. From listening to parents who have attempted and failed with this method, they say that the reason they gave up is that, contrary to the claims that their baby will not cry, there is usually some degree of crying involved. That, along with the fact that this approach can take up to two weeks or even longer to work, is the reason that I believe so many parents give up because they simply cannot cope with night after night of crying.

I am not going to promise that using my plan will not involve some crying, but what I can say is that any crying will be kept to the minimum and that within a few nights your baby should be settling to sleep with only a short spell of crying down. Please refer to page 160 so that you understand the difference between crying down and crying up.

ONE-WEEK PLAN FOR DITCHING THE DUMMY

DAY ONE

- Eliminate the dummy at nap times by taking him out in his buggy for a walk or in the car.
- He can still be given the dummy at bedtime and during the night.

DAYS TWO TO THREE

- Implement the later bedtime described on (page 124) so that he is only given the dummy at the 10pm feed or in the night.

DAYS FOUR TO FIVE

- By this stage your baby will only have been having the dummy at the late bedtime and when he wakes in the night, therefore now is the time to eliminate the dummy completely.
- Bring his bedtime back to 7pm and settle him in his cot sleepy but awake and shush and pat him to sleep (see page 155).
- If he gets very upset he can be picked up and calmed down, but it is important that you put him back in his cot before he goes to sleep.
- Each time he wakes in the night, use the same approach: shush and pat him back to sleep, only lifting him out of the cot if he is getting really upset. Remember that he must be settled back in the cot sleepy but awake.

DAYS SIX TO SEVEN

- By day seven I usually find that most babies are settling within a few minutes of waking by being shushed and patted, therefore now is the time to allow him to self-settle.
- Place him in the cot sleepy but awake, and for a minute or so gently stroke or pat his tummy and say, 'Night, sleepy time,' and then leave the room.
- At this stage you should be able to implement crying-down time, as described on page 160.
- Most babies will settle within a few minutes of crying down, although I do find that a few babies will fight sleep and take a little longer to settle.

7

Co-sleeping to Cot Sleeping

Many of the parents who come to me for help on moving their baby from sleeping in their bed to happily sleeping in their own cot have chosen to co-sleep from day one. Others have ended up co-sleeping by accident. During a bout of illness parents often take their restless baby into bed with them in desperation or, when babies are waking up multiple times in the night, an exhausted parent will end up taking the baby into their bed. It is not really so important *why* you ended up sharing your bed with your baby; what is more important is how you transfer your baby from your bed to their own bed, with the least possible distress. Unlike some of the other sleep problems covered in this book, which can be relatively simple to resolve, getting a baby who has been used to the comfort of sleeping with you in your bed happily settling in their own bed, is not quite so straightforward. However, with careful planning and a great deal of patience it most certainly can be done.

Time and time again I get parents coming to me saying that they have tried to follow a 'gentle' or one of the many 'no cry' sleep plans to resolve their baby's sleep problems, only to give up within a couple of nights, or even worse within hours of the first night, because their baby was crying so hysterically, often for hours on end, despite following the plan to the letter. I am not going to promise you that transitioning your baby from your bed to his own will be easy or that there will not be some upset or tears, but what I can say is that if you follow my plan to the letter you should not end up with your baby screaming for hours on end.

What makes my sleep plan different from so many of the others that are available is that I advise parents to do things in stages. This is particularly important when you are implementing a co-sleeping to cot sleeping plan. Co-sleeping usually goes hand in hand with assisting to sleep, by feeding, rocking or giving the dummy. If you were using all of these sleep props to get your baby to sleep along with taking him into your bed and he then slept soundly all night, you probably would not be reading this book. The reality is that if your baby is co-sleeping he will more than likely have at least one, if not all, of the other sleep problems mentioned above.

The success of my co-sleeping to cot sleeping plan is that the problem you address first when transitioning your baby from your bed to his cot is getting rid of the sleep aids that help assist your baby to sleep (the main ones being feeding, rocking and the dummy). However, at this point I would not advise you attempt to get rid of any middle-of-the-night feeds during the cot transition, even if your baby is older than six months and no longer really needs them. Night feeds will be much easier to eliminate once your baby is happily self-settling and sleeping in his cot. During the transition period, night feeds can actually be of help in getting your baby to self-settle easier in the cot. In addition, offering a feed at this stage is much more preferable than offering the dummy or a cuddle, as there is less chance of the baby waking up an hour later if they have had a good feed. The only rule to remember when feeding your baby in the night is to ensure that you do not feed him to sleep. Within a few nights of following the plan you should find that your baby is happy self-settling in his cot and sleeping for longer spells in between feeds, and it is at this stage that you can then look to eliminate night feeds using the core night method described on page 163.

Before you even consider transitioning your baby from your bed to his cot there are some important factors that you have to take into consideration. Successful transition will be dependent on several things:

- You and your partner must be in complete agreement that getting your baby to sleep independently in his own bed is what you both really want.
- During the transition from your bed to your baby's cot, you will have to also deal with any other sleep props that your baby has become reliant upon. It is no good transferring your baby to his own cot, only to still continue rocking, feeding or giving him the dummy to get him to sleep. In my experience, parents who continue to use these sleep aids will, within several nights, end up taking their baby back into bed with them.

- Finally, and this is probably one of the most important rules when transferring your baby into his own bed: you must be consistent. It is pointless going through several nights of getting your baby to sleep happily in his own bed to end up two or three weeks down the line thinking it is fine to take him into bed occasionally. There are no half measures when transitioning your baby from your bed to his cot – if it is to be successful it is either all or nothing.

If you and your partner are both in absolute agreement that you want your baby sleeping independently in his own bed, the next move is to prepare a proper transition plan:

- One of the main keys to ensuring that the plan will work is to choose the right time. It is not advisable to start the plan if your baby is ill, if you or your partner are going through a stressful time at work or if you have grandparents or visitors coming to stay. Equally you want to make sure that your diary is clear of evening social events for at least a week.

- Ideally I would recommend that you start the plan on a Friday night, as the first two nights are most likely to be the worst in terms of tiredness, with you being awake for possibly a considerable part of the night.

- If you have older children and are concerned about them being woken in the night, if possible see if they can have a sleepover with grandparents or at a friend's house on the first night you implement the plan, or even for two nights.

- Decide which one of you is going to do the settling in the evening and the middle of the night. Ideally, especially on the first night, I always think that it is best if the same parent settles the baby at both of these times. I think it can be very confusing for the baby when parents are taking turns at settling. If you think that this will not be possible, you should certainly aim for one parent to do the whole early evening settling and the other the whole of the middle-of-the-night settling, rather than swapping over in the middle of a settling period.

- Be prepared that for the first two or three nights your baby's sleeping may actually get worse before it gets better. Sometimes the first couple of nights may go really well and then suddenly the third night can be very difficult. This is quite a common pattern, so please do not get despondent if this happens.

ONE-WEEK PLAN FOR TRANSITIONING FROM BED TO COT

Because it is recommended that babies sleep in their parents' room for the first six months, the co-sleeping to cot plan is divided into two sections – the first for young babies under six months old and the second for babies over six months. With a baby over six months, if you still have the cot in your room, I would recommend that you use this plan to not only transition him from your bed to his cot, but also from your room to his own room.

Birth to six months

For babies of this age, I would advise following the 'assisting-to-sleep method', as set out on page 157. This technique aims to get the baby used to sleeping at regular times and is very useful for young babies that don't sleep well in the evening and have ended up sleeping in their parents' bed. Once your baby is sleeping well using this method you can then move on from any sleep associations using the relevant advice in the earlier chapters of this book.

Six to twelve months

The first step of the plan is to actually delay the time you put your baby to bed for the first three nights. By delaying the bedtime it actually reduces the length of time you expect your baby to sleep in his cot, which will lessen the time he has to get upset about going into the cot, plus the amount of sleep that you may lose during the night getting him to settle in his cot. It may be that, if you have been doing planned co-sleeping, your baby is already not going to bed until you do, so that will in fact make the plan easier to follow. However, if your baby is settling in his bed in the evening and then coming into your bed in the middle of the night or the early hours of the morning, I would recommend that you delay bedtime. I know that this may seem a little daunting, but it is only for a few nights and it will help avoid the problem of your baby waking up really early and you having the problems of trying to get him back to sleep around 6am. Remember what I said earlier: that consistency is the key to resolving this problem – you can't not take your baby into your bed in the middle of the night and then suddenly take him into bed at 5.30 or 6am because it is too near his usual wake-up time. Delaying the bedtime for the first three nights will help resolve this problem.

The aim of the first three nights is to get your baby settling and sleeping well in his cot without any sleep aid, such as rocking and giving the dummy. Don't worry about night feeds at this stage, as a baby who has just had a milk feed should be easier to settle than one who hasn't. Getting rid of the night feeds will quickly be resolved once your baby is settling and sleeping well in his cot (see Chapter 3).

With the later bedtime, I would aim to have your baby asleep somewhere between 9 and 10pm, which will mean that you would start the bath and bedtime routine around 8.30pm. If your baby is used to settling around 7pm, I would recommend that you alter his routine slightly so that his tea and evening milk feed come later. Please see the guidelines below on how to do this:

- Small snack and milk feed around 4.30pm to replace normal solids given around 5pm.
- Instead of doing the bath at your usual time, I would recommend that you extend play time and then prepare your baby for a short nap near to his usual bedtime, so that he can stay up later without getting overtired.
- I would not recommend that you attempt to put him in his cot at this time, as it is important that the right sleep associations are in place on the first night of the plan. If you are concerned about him not sleeping at this time, it is fine to assist him as long as you do not put him in the cot. If need be, and weather permitting, either you or your partner can take him out in the buggy to get him to sleep. If needed, even a short trip in the car is fine – the main thing is to get your baby to sleep for ideally an hour, so that when he does wake he can stay happily awake for a further couple of hours.

- When he wakes from this nap you should give him his normal tea.
- It is important to calculate how long you think he can stay awake happily for after he wakes, so that you can decide what time you are going to implement his bath and bedtime routine. For example, if he falls asleep at 6.45pm and wakes up at 7.45pm, and you know he can stay awake happily for a couple of hours, I would be aiming that he should be in his cot no later than 9.30pm. Therefore, your evening would look a little like the following:

7.45pm	Solids
8.15pm	Quiet playtime before the bath
8.45pm	Bath and massage
9.15pm	Milk feed in his nursery – he should not be allowed to get sleepy on the bottle or breast
9.45pm	He must be placed in the cot sleepy but still awake

NIGHT ONE

I would recommend that for the first two to three nights you stay in the room with your baby while he settles to sleep. I know that some methods recommend leaving the room and checking every five to ten minutes, but I really would not recommend this approach at this stage. Instead I would advise that you sit beside your baby's cot so that you can pat and shush him if he becomes upset (see page 155 for more on the shush-pat technique). If he is nearer a year old he may keep sitting or standing up. Each time he does this you should lay him down and shush and pat until he calms down. Some babies will get themselves off to sleep within 10 to 20 minutes; with others it can take an hour or even longer.

If you find your baby gets really distressed, it is fine to pick him up and calm him down, as long as you get him in the cot before he falls asleep. When calming him down, try to use a position where you can see his face, such as lying across you as opposed to putting him over your shoulder where you cannot see if he is dozing off to sleep.

When he wakes in the night, try not to rush to him if he is just tossing and turning or grumbling. However, if he is starting to cry up (see page 161) I would attend to him before he gets into a state.

There is no benefit to him being allowed to get into a distressed state on the first night you are trying to get him to sleep without you next to him. If it is only an hour or two since he fed and you are persistent with the shushing and patting, you should manage to get him back to sleep within 45 minutes to an hour. However, if he sleeps for more than three or four hours, I would advise that you offer him a milk feed, so that he needs less assistance to sleep. This is especially so if he has been used to feeding in the night anyway.

Each time he wakes in the night you repeat the same procedure of shushing and patting and laying him down, remembering that if he cries up and is getting hysterical you can pick him up and comfort him as long as you get him back in the cot sleepy, but awake. If he sleeps a further three to four hours, he can then be offered another milk feed if you are having problems settling him.

Regardless of what he has done in the night, I would strongly urge that you wake him up no later than 7am. Leaving him to sleep longer in the morning could delay how long he takes to settle on the second night.

DAY TWO

During the day I would not recommend that you put him in his cot for his naps. Because of the limited timeframe you have to get him to sleep, if he does not settle and then you have to get him up because he is due a feed anyway, it could send the wrong sleep associations. I would recommend that you take him out in the buggy or car for his daytime naps.

NIGHT TWO

Repeat the procedure exactly as you did on night one, but this time allow slightly longer between shushing and patting him, without allowing him to cry up, to see if he is trying to settle himself. Like the first night, if he is going three to four hours between wakings, you can feed him if he does not settle quickly. Remember, the aim is still to get him to self-settle without being fed to sleep or being rocked or given the dummy to sleep.

DAY THREE

If you feel you are making progress with the nights and he is settling fairly quickly in the night, you can now try putting him in his cot for his longest nap of the day. You should use the same procedure as you have in the night, but I would recommend that you only attempt to get him through one sleep cycle. Trying to get him through a second sleep cycle could result in him getting really upset and, as you don't have the same length of time to resettle him as you do in the night, it would be best to just get him up if he begins to cry up when he comes into his second sleep cycle. Obviously, he would need to have a short nap in the late afternoon, but, like the morning nap, I would recommend that you take him out in the buggy or car for this.

NIGHT THREE

On night three I would gradually begin to reduce the amount of shushing and patting that you are doing. You can still stay in the room until he falls asleep, but lengthen the time that you are next to the cot physically shushing him. Instead, sit on a chair a little distance from the cot and verbally reassure him that you are still here. Use the same simple phrase 'shush, shush, sleepy time' or similar.

On night three you should also aim to reduce any milk he may be having in the night. For example, if he has been having milk at 2 and 5am, then try to settle him back by shushing or patting or, if needed, 60–90ml (2–3oz) of milk. If he is less than nine months it would probably be best to give this in a bottle; if he is between nine and twelve months, a soft spouted beaker; and for breast-fed babies who do not take a bottle, a beaker works well.

DAY FOUR

If your baby is settling fairly quickly when you put him down in the evening and when he wakes in the night, you can now put him in his cot for both of his daytime naps should you wish. On day four you should also start to bring his bedtime forward by 30 minutes, which means you will need to reduce the early evening nap by 20 minutes.

NIGHT FOUR

On night four you should start to gradually retreat from the bedroom. Your baby could well protest and he may actually take longer to settle this evening, but it is important that you start to reduce the amount of help you give him with settling. I would recommend that you stay in his room for 10 minutes sitting on a chair and verbally reassuring him every few minutes. You should then leave the room for a couple of minutes, but remain right outside the door, verbally reassuring him. You then repeat the procedure of two or three minutes outside the room and five to ten minutes inside the room. At this stage you really must try to resist picking him up – try if possible to reassure him in the cot. If he keeps pulling himself up in the cot, you should keep lying him back down. You may have to do this many times, until he eventually gets himself off to sleep. Whatever time he fed last at on night three, aim to feed him 30 minutes later than that. If he only fed once in the night last night, then aim to replace that one feed with a small drink of water. However, if he wakes around 5.30 or 6am I would certainly feed him then if it seems that he is not going to go back to sleep fairly quickly.

DAY FIVE

You want to bring his bedtime forward by a further 45 minutes this evening, so I would reduce his early evening nap by a further 20 minutes.

NIGHT FIVE

On night five you continue with the checking method and verbally reassuring him, but extend the time you are outside the room from two to five minutes and shorten the time you are in the room and how often you are reassuring him.

DAY SIX

By the sixth night your baby should be settling much more quickly in the evening, waking up less in the night and settling back very quickly. I would aim to settle him in bed at the time you have decided is going to be his regular bedtime. Bring his tea back to the normal time and aim for his bath and bedtime routine at the normal time.

NIGHT SIX

Once you have settled your baby in his bed you should leave the room immediately and try to wait at least 15 to 20 minutes before going in to settle him. Obviously, if he is getting himself in a state and crying up, then you can check him sooner than the 20 minutes, but if possible do try to wait before going in. You can verbally reassure him from the doorway, but it is important that you keep gradually extending the time between the verbal reassurances that you give him.

DAY SEVEN

Today your baby should follow his normal routine and aim for the same bedtime as night six. If he settled within 15 to 20 minutes last night, once you leave the room you should aim to wait a little longer before going back to reassure him, and this should only be done if he is crying up. You can continue to verbally reassure him from outside the room but you still need to continue extending the time before reassuring him.

In the night when he wakes, unless he woke up crying really hard, you should allow him time to resettle himself. I usually find that by this time most babies will settle themselves back to sleep after 10 to 20 minutes of on-and-off grizzling. Occasionally I have had a baby who took slightly longer to settle back, but by the seventh night I certainly was not having to keep going in and out of the room, or offering a feed in the middle of the night. However, if your baby wakes nearer to 6am I would certainly offer a night feed for a further week or two to ensure that he sleeps to nearer 7am.

It can be very hard leaving your baby to cry, for even the shortest of times, particularly if you have been used to cuddling and sleeping right next to him. But try to remember that the reason that you are doing this is to help your baby become an independent and happy sleeper. Establishing healthy sleep habits from the first year will help your baby grow up into a confident and happy child who enjoys a full night's sleep and is therefore able to cope with the many challenges he faces during his growing-up years. In my experience of advising thousands of parents, the first few nights are the worst, but by the end of the week you should be well on the way to having a contented little baby who is happy to go in his cot.

8

General Sleep Techniques

Throughout this book I've suggested a number of gentle plans and sleep-training methods that you can use to overcome specific sleeping problems and associations. This chapter contains the key techniques that can be used in many circumstances.

Before you consider any sleep-training methods, it is important to consider what is suitable for your baby's age.

BIRTH TO SIX MONTHS

Although many baby experts advise parents not to use any sleep-training methods until their baby is over six months old it is my belief that waiting this long can mean poor sleep patterns and associations become fully ingrained and far more difficult to resolve. Babies who have learned the wrong sleep associations will be unable to get back to sleep unaided and will need whatever methods the parents use to assist them to sleep, be it feeding, rocking or the dummy. Some babies may need all three comforts before dropping back off to sleep. These babies are very unlikely to learn to sleep through the night until they are much older (in my experience this is usually between the second and third year) and typically continue to wake up several times a night. With sleep training it is your aim to allow your baby to learn to go to sleep unassisted, and it is important to remember that this will prevent much greater upset and more crying if your baby is waking in the night from a light sleep not knowing how to go back to sleep by himself.

Many sleep-training techniques are not suitable for babies under six months old. The only techniques in this chapter I would recommend for this age are the shush-pat technique (page 155), the assisting-to-sleep routine (page 157) and crying down (page 160).

BABIES OVER SIX MONTHS

With babies between six months and one year of age, waking in the night is often due to a mixture of hunger and association, caused by a lack of structure in the baby's feeding and sleeping. With toddlers and babies who have already got into seriously bad sleeping habits, the following sleep-training techniques will need to be used along with the advice for sleeping and feeding requirements in earlier chapters.

If an older baby or toddler has learned the wrong sleep associations and needs to be rocked, cuddled or fed to sleep, then it is likely that some degree of controlled crying will have to be implemented if sleep training is to be successful. However, if these children are still feeding in the night, it is advisable to implement the core night method (see page 163) first so that you can be confident that your baby or toddler is not crying through genuine hunger.

Controlled crying is a very effective way to train babies over six months but should always be used as a last resort, when all other methods have failed. One of the main reasons that controlled crying fails for so many parents is that a vicious circle arises in which the baby continues to feed in the night and does not eat enough during the day, so he is genuinely hungry in the night. The core night method and gradually reducing your baby's milk feed in the night should see an increase in his appetite during the day.

I would not recommend that a parent attempts controlled crying until they see an increase in the amount of food their child is eating during the day. Dr Richard Ferber, author of *Solve Your Child's Sleep Problems*, advises gradually eliminating night feeds for older babies and toddlers who are still feeding in the night. If waking continues, he recommends controlled crying to break the habit.

KEY SLEEP TECHNIQUES

Most of the methods that follow are very gentle and involve very little crying. Over the last few years I have successfully used these gentle methods to solve the problems of thousands of babies. However, occasionally I have had to deal with a baby where the habits have become so deep-rooted that I had no option but to use controlled crying. I have always believed that controlled crying should only be used as a last resort to solve problems, when all other methods have failed. If you decide that a tougher form of sleep training is needed for your baby, it is essential that he has a check-up with your GP to confirm that there are no medical reasons why you should not attempt controlled crying.

It is important not to confuse controlled crying with crying down. To have a better understanding of the difference between controlled crying and crying down, please carefully read page 160–3.

Shush-pat technique

The technique of 'shushing' and patting your baby has been used to help babies calm down and drift off to sleep since time immemorial. It is a great technique for babies from birth, especially when you are trying to break free from sleep associations such as rocking or feeding to sleep.

- Lay your baby in his basket or cot. For babies under six months, you should position him on his side.

With an older baby of six months or more, I find it better to move him onto his tummy, holding him down with one hand so you can pat with the other.

- If your baby will not calm down in his cot, you can start this technique with him in your arms or over your shoulder, and then move him to his cot once he has calmed down.

- Whisper 'shush, shush' while you rhythmically and steadily pat the centre of his back. The patting should be quite firm, about the pace of clock or heartbeat. Make sure you do not shush directly into his ear.

- Continue to shush-pat for a few minutes after he has calmed down, gradually slowing down the patting and stopping the shushing. Then move away from the cot to see if your baby can settle himself to sleep.

- Some babies will get themselves off to sleep within 10 to 20 minutes; with others it can take an hour or even longer.

- If he wakes and cries, you can continue shushing and patting again.

- For babies that are not yet rolling, you will need to roll him onto his back once he is asleep, as

research has shown this to be the safest sleep
position – see page 106–7 for more on this).

Assisting-to-sleep routine

The 'assisting-to-sleep routine' is a technique that
I use with very young babies who are unsettled in
the evening and refusing to settle in their cots. It can
also be used for very young babies who have become
used to not sleeping well in the evening and who have
ended up sleeping in their parents' bed. It is a form of
sleep prop but it is only used in a structured way for
a very short time, so please don't worry that this will
make things worse. Provided you are getting your
baby's feeding and sleeping structured properly, then
using the assisting-to-sleep routine for a short time
will be the final step you need to take to get your
baby settling well.

The aim of the assisting-to-sleep routine is to get
your baby used to sleeping at regular times during
naps and in the evening. Once your baby is used
to sleeping at the same times for several days, you
should find that you can settle him in his bed with
the minimum of fuss.

For this method to work it is important that it is done consistently and by only one parent.

- During stage one of the routine, and for at least three days, do not attempt to put your baby in his bed at nap times or early evening. Instead, one parent should lie in a quiet room with him and cuddle him throughout the whole of the sleep time.

- Try to ensure that your baby is held in the crook of your arm, rather than lying across your chest. If he is older than two months and is no longer swaddled, it may help to use your right hand to hold both his hands across his chest; in this way, he will not wave his arms around and risk getting upset.

- It is important that the same person is with him during the allocated sleep time, and that you do not hand him back and forth, or walk from room to room.

- Once he is sleeping soundly for three days in a row at the recommended times, you should then progress on to the second stage and try to settle him in his bed.

- It is important to sit right next to his bed, so you can hold his hands across his chest and comfort him.

- On the fourth night, hold both his hands until he is asleep, and on the fifth night hold only one of his hands across his chest until he is asleep.

- By the sixth night you should find that you can put him down sleepy but awake in his bed, checking him every two or three minutes until he falls asleep. Do not try to settle him in his bed unless he has been sleeping soundly in your arms for at least three nights.

- Once he is settling within 10 minutes for several nights, you should try leaving him to self-settle using the crying-down method described on page 160.

- It will help your baby get used to being happy in his bed if you put him in it for short spells during the day, when he is fully awake, with a small book or toy to look at.

- For the lunchtime nap, if you prefer, you can take your baby out for a nap in his buggy. The important thing is to try to be consistent; the lunchtime nap should be in the buggy or in the home, but do

not switch from one to the other midway through
the nap.

After several nights of your baby sleeping well in
the evening using the assisting-to-sleep routine, you
can then start to eliminate whichever sleep props you
are using to get your baby to sleep. For feeding to
sleep please refer to Chapter 3, for rocking to sleep,
see Chapter 4 and for eliminating the use of the
dummy please refer to Chapter 6.

Crying down

Provided a baby has been well fed and is ready
to sleep, I believe he should be allowed to settle
himself. When an overtired baby is going to sleep he
often cries a little before settling. 'Crying down' is
a term used by Dr Brian Symon, aka 'the Babysleep
Doctor' author of *Silent Nights* and a senior lecturer
in general practice at the University of Adelaide, to
describe the pattern of crying when an overtired
baby is going to sleep.

Crying down, he says, is the reverse of 'crying up',
with crying up being the description of a baby waking

up from a good sleep and starting to demand a feed. Crying up starts with silence. The baby is asleep, he then wakes. His first sounds are soft, gentle and subtle. After a minute or two of being left alone, the baby begins to cry. He will cry for a short spell, then go quiet for a short spell. If he is left, the crying starts again but louder. The crying gradually increases in volume, with the gaps between cries becoming shorter until the baby is emitting a continuous loud bellow.

Crying down is the reverse of that picture. The overtired baby will start to bellow loudly when put him down to sleep and the reverse pattern begins. In my experience the process of crying down to sleep takes between 10 and 20 minutes. The more overtired the baby is, the louder and longer he will cry. Dr Symon stresses that this technique will only work if the baby is allowed to settle himself to sleep. Crying down can be particularly helpful when feeding problems have been resolved and a baby has only mild sleep-association problems or has difficulty falling asleep because he is overtired or overstimulated. It also works for babies who fight sleep.

Although it is very difficult to listen to a young baby cry himself to sleep, it will prevent serious sleep problems in the future. Parents who find the crying difficult to ignore are advised to wait 10 minutes before going in to him. They can then enter and reassure the baby with a soothing touch or quiet voice. Reassurance must be kept to a maximum of one to two minutes. Parents should then wait a further 10–15 minutes before returning. For this technique to work, it is essential that the baby is not picked up and that he is allowed to settle by himself in his cot.

Dr Symon believes that parents who do not allow their overtired baby to get himself off to sleep are creating long-term sleep problems. His beliefs have recently been confirmed by research at Oxford University. They conclude that a 20-minute 'winding down' bedtime routine, coupled with ignoring crying for gradually increasing intervals, is an effective way of dealing with babies and children who resist sleep.

Parents who are not prepared to leave their baby to cry for 10–20 minutes usually end up resorting to feeding, rocking or giving a dummy to induce sleep. This can often take up to two hours, resulting in exhausted parents and the baby waking up when he comes into his light sleep looking for the same inducement to get back to sleep again. It is my belief that, in the long-term, allowing your baby to develop the wrong sleep associations and therefore denying him the sound night's sleep he needs in order to develop both mentally and physically is a worse option than hearing him cry for a short while.

Crying down with a baby under six weeks usually lasts between five and ten minutes, although with some babies who have become overtired and fight sleep it can last up to 20 minutes. Provided all the baby's needs have been met, he will normally learn how to settle himself to sleep within a few nights, although some babies do continue to cry down at bedtime for several weeks. However, the time they cry usually gets progressively less.

If you are breast-feeding, I would always advise that you offer your baby a top-up of expressed milk before attempting crying down, to be 100 per cent sure that hunger is not the reason he is not settling.

The core night method

The core night method has been used for many years by maternity nurses and parents who believe in routine. It works on the principle that once a baby sleeps for one longer spell in the night, he should never again be fed during the hours slept in the course of the core night. If he wakes during those hours, he should be left for a few minutes to settle himself back to sleep. If he refuses to settle, then other methods apart from feeding should be used to settle him.

There are different approaches for the other methods. Beatrice Hollyer and Lucy Smith, authors of *Sleep: The Easy Way to Peaceful Nights*, recommend patting, offering a dummy or giving a sip of water. However, I must stress that it is now recommended that babies under six months are not given water (see page 166 for more on this). Attention should be kept to the minimum while reassuring the baby that you are there. They claim that following this approach will, within days, have your baby sleeping at least the hours of his first core night. It also teaches the baby the most important two sleep skills: how to go to sleep and how to go back to sleep after surfacing from a non-REM (non-rapid eye movement) sleep. Dr Brian Symon recommends a similar approach for babies over six weeks: for babies who are putting on a good amount of weight each week but still waking at 3am, give the shortest feed possible that will allow him to settle.

Before embarking on this method, the following points should be read carefully to make sure that your baby really is capable of going for a longer spell in the night:

- These methods should never be used with a very small baby or a baby who is not gaining weight. A baby not gaining weight should always be seen by a doctor.
- The above methods should only be used if your baby is gaining weight steadily, and if you are sure that his last feed is substantial enough to help him sleep for the longer stretch in the night.
- The main sign that a baby is ready to cut down on a night feed is a regular weight gain and the reluctance to feed, or tendency to feed less, at 7am.
- The aim of using any of the above methods is gradually to increase the length of time your baby can go from his last feed and not to eliminate the night feeds all in one go.

- The core night method can be used if, over three or four nights, a baby has shown signs that he is capable of sleeping for a longer stretch.

- If your baby does not settle within 20 minutes of using the core night method, then he should be given a big enough feed for a further week or so to get him through to nearer 7am, before trying again. There is no advantage to having your baby awake for lengthy periods in the night, as it will only cause him to need more sleep during the day. Too much sleep in the day will only cause him to be more unsettled in the night.

- The method can be used to try to reduce the number of times a demand-fed baby is fed in the night and to encourage him to go for a longer stretch between feeds, or after his last daytime feed.

Offering water

For many years it was recommended that a small drink of cool boiled water (around 30ml/1oz) could be offered to a baby aged between eight and twelve weeks who may be waking up at around 2–3am out of habit and not hunger. In my original books I only advised this if a baby took the water and then settled back to sleep for a couple of hours. Recently the advice on what age to give water has changed and it is recommended that babies are not given water before six months of age.

If your baby is over six months of age and waking up in the night through habit and not hunger, it is fine to offer 30ml (1oz) or so of cool boiled water in the hope that he gets back to sleep. However, it is pointless to keep offering water at this time if your baby refuses to settle back to sleep quickly or wakes up again after 30–40 minutes. If you persist with offering water over several nights with an unsettled baby, you will actually be encouraging your baby to sleep badly in the night, which is the opposite of what you really want. Night feeds are easier to eliminate when a baby feeds quickly and settles back to sleep until the morning, rather than when a baby who is awake on and off during the night is offered water, the dummy or cuddles to get back to sleep. However, it is important also to look at your baby's daytime feeding and improve on that so he does not wake up in the night due to genuine hunger. For more on this, see page 26.

CONTROLLED CRYING

The controlled crying method is likely to be more successful if used at each of the baby's sleep times. While this method does teach a baby or toddler how to get to sleep on his own, it can be difficult to endure and can fail because parents get very distressed listening to their child cry for lengthy periods of time. They resort to picking him up after 30–40 minutes and rocking him to sleep, which usually creates an even worse sleep problem. The baby soon learns that if he cries long and hard enough, he will be picked up. I understand that it can be very distressing to listen to your child crying for any length of time. However, if done properly, this method will improve even the worst sleeping problems within days. In my experience, with older babies and toddlers the problem is normally resolved within a week. For controlled crying to be successful it is essential that the child learns to settle himself to sleep, no matter how long it takes.

The basic rules for controlled crying are as follows:

NIGHT ONE

It is always best to start controlled crying in the evening on the first day. The same procedure should be carried out no matter how many times the baby or toddler wakes in the night. The following day it is important that you stick to the routine appropriate for your baby or toddler's age and that you use the same procedure when settling him for daytime naps as you use in the evening.

- Decide on a regular time to start the bedtime routine and stick to it. Allow at least one hour for the bath, milk feed and settling.
- Settle your baby or child in his bed before he gets too sleepy. Kiss him goodnight and leave the room.
- Allow a minimum of 5–10 minutes of crying before returning to reassure him. Reassurance should be kept to the minimum. You can stroke him or say

'shush, shush', but he must not be picked up. Leave the room after two minutes even if he continues to cry.

- After the first half hour, the time between visits should be increased by 5–10 minutes each time, to 15–20 minutes between visits.

- Continue with the checking plan every 15–20 minutes until the baby or toddler falls asleep. Reassurance should still be kept to a minimum of no more than two minutes and he must not be lifted out of the cot.

- If your baby wakes in the night, continue to follow the same plan as for the evening, gradually increasing the time between visits, until you are going in every 15–20 minutes.

DAY TWO

- For the daytime naps it is important that you start where you left off in the night. Wait at least 20 minutes before checking your baby or toddler and continue to keep visits to his room to a maximum of two minutes, with the minimum of reassurance.

- If your baby does not fall asleep until nearer the time the routine states that he is meant to be getting up, allow him 10–15 minutes at the morning nap and 30–40 minutes at the lunchtime nap; this way he will not end up sleeping after 3pm in the day. If your baby is very tired he may need a short nap of 15 or 20 minutes in the late afternoon if he is to get through until bedtime without becoming overtired.

NIGHT TWO

- The second evening follow the same settling procedure as the first night, but this time wait 20–25 minutes before returning to the nursery. During visits on the second night you can reassure your baby by saying 'shush, shush', but do not stroke or touch him.
- If your baby is still crying on and off after the first hour, the time between visits should be increased to 30–40 minutes.
- If he wakes in the night, you should wait 40 minutes before checking him, and you should not speak to or stroke him. Reduce the time in the room to one minute providing he is not hysterical.

DAY THREE

- By the third day, the majority of babies will be settling themselves at all sleep times within 10–20 minutes and there is no need to check on them.

- If your baby backtracks at one of the sleep times and you have to go back to checking him, start off with checking him every 15–20 minutes and increase the interval until you are back to 40–50 minutes.

- By the third day aim to achieve a time of no less than 15–20 minutes. Do not go back to checking every 5–10 minutes, as this usually results in the baby getting more upset by your visits.

- Once your baby has done a few days of settling within 20 minutes, you should be able to use the crying-down method (see page 160) for getting him off to sleep at naps or in the evening. Within a couple of weeks the majority of babies will be going to sleep without any fuss at all.

Conclusion

Over the last 20 years through my consultancy I have helped thousands of parents resolve their babies' sleep problems using the gentle methods outlined in this book. When parents come to me struggling with how to deal with their baby's sleep problems, I always stress that whilst it is important to understand why the sleep problems have developed, it is equally important not to dwell on the reasons why, but instead to move forward and take control of the problem. It is all too easy to keep delaying dealing with a problem in the hope that the baby will eventually start to sleep better naturally. In my experience the types of problems covered in this book rarely resolve themselves. Sleep deprivation affects not only the baby but the whole family and the sooner a healthy sleep pattern is established the sooner calm and happiness will be restored within the family.

To get the best out of the methods in this book I advise that both parents should read the book and then agree upon a plan that you think will work best for your baby. I usually advise that parents start the plan on a Thursday or Friday, as the first few days are usually the most difficult, it is good to have no work pressures whilst implementing the plan. Remember that the guidelines in this book are exactly just that, if your instinct is to stay on a particular stage of the plan a few days longer than I recommend, then that is fine.

You may also find it helpful to check out my website www.contentedbaby.com where you can access dozens of the case studies that I have worked on, along with support from other parents who have had similar problems. If you feel you would like professional help in resolving your problems, please do not hesitate in contacting cbc@contentedbaby. com.

Index